D0197125

Praise for *The Big Fat Truth* and JD Roth

"To lose weight for good, you need to become a beast—a beast who crushes your workouts, who can outsmart temptation, and who has shed the fat in your head. On *The Biggest Loser,* JD Roth was the guy who could wake the beast within anyone. With *The Big Fat Truth,* he can wake the weight-loss beast in you."

—JILLIAN MICHAELS, The Biggest Loser

"JD Roth has a passion for making this world a better place and a unique experience helping people change their interaction with food. His ideas are as original—and professional—as any I have heard on this important question. His views are inspiring, and they will help you lose weight forever."

—T. COLIN CAMPBELL, PhD,
bestselling author of The China Study

"A lot of people who want to lose weight think food is the enemy. I've devoted years to combating that mind-set, introducing America to real, healthy, comfort food. JD Roth will shatter it in minutes—and show you how to slay the mental hang-ups that are the real enemy of lasting weight loss and absurdly good health and happiness."

—ROCCO DISPIRITO,
chef, TV host, and author of Now Eat This! and The Pound-a-Day Diet

"JD is a reality engineer who possesses the gift to create the real we all want!"

—ASHTON KUTCHER

"On camera, you see incredible stories of transformation . . . but off camera is where the magic happens. Yes, you need to diet and exercise to lose weight, but making the heart and mind connection—with yourself and with others—is what will change your life forever. No one knows how to make that connection better than JD Roth."

—CHRIS AND HEIDI POWELL, Extreme Weight Loss

"I respect JD Roth's total commitment and passion for helping people live their best life possible. Through his time with *The Biggest Loser* he learned it was not just about a physical transformation but an emotional shift that helped facilitate that external change. So whether you need to lose 10 pounds or 110 pounds, *The Big Fat Truth* will be a helpful resource of information and inspiration."

—GABBY REECE,
volleyball player, sports announcer, model, and author

"JD Roth throws out a life line to those who want to lose weight. He's a powerful compassionate ally whose tough love approach will absolutely help you shed extra pounds. *The Big Fat Truth* is your answer to a healthier, lighter you!"

—MING-NA WEN, actress and founder of WENever

"JD Roth will cheer louder for you, fight harder for you and believe more in you than you may even do for yourself…. [W]hile reading his book you will feel his inspiration, devotion, commitment, and passion to make our bodies less heavy and our hearts more full."

—IDAN RAVIN,
author of the nationally acclaimed *The Hoops Whisperer*
and a world-renowned trainer who has worked with superstars such as
Stephen Curry, James Harden, Chris Paul, and Carmelo Anthony

"JD Roth embodies empathy and compassion, two qualities that are exceptionally rare is this industry. His lessons and examples make this book a must-read."

—TIM GUNN, *Project Runway*

"This book isn't about weight loss; it's about life gain. JD is the ultimate coach. He encourages, believes, motivates, and, above all, loves those who don't love themselves. Thank you, JD, for giving the best of yourself to help others."

—CHARISSA THOMPSON, co-host on *Fox NFL* and *Extra*

"I had the opportunity to work with JD for many years on *The Biggest Loser*. This is definitely a man that thinks outside the box. He is passionate about what he does and he believes with his whole heart that we all can and, more importantly, all *deserve* to live the life that we are meant to live."

—BOB HARPER, *The Biggest Loser*

"JD's unparalleled positive energy is contagious. He motivates and inspires even the most pessimistic, and has bottled his message of positivity in this book!"

—HARLEY PASTERNAK, MSc,
New York Times bestselling author of
The Body Reset Diet, 5-Factor Diet, and *5-Factor Fitness*

"Though the process of weight-loss is a complex one, and controversy may exist in the medical and nutritional worlds about how to best accomplish this goal, one thing is certain: it all starts with the mind-body connection. No one knows this better than JD Roth. If he could write a prescription for that, it would be 'inspiration: take one daily; repeat indefinitely'!"

—JENNIFER L. ASHTON, MD, FACOG,
ABC News Senior Medical Contributor on
Good Morning America and co-host of *The Doctors*

"JD has a way of finding the best in everyone. With his book, he'll help you find the best in yourself!"

—DOLVETT QUINCE, *The Biggest Loser*

The

BIG FAT
TRUTH

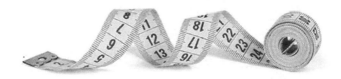

Behind-the-Scenes Secrets
to **Losing Weight** and
Gaining the Inner Strength
to Transform Your Life

JD ROTH

Foreword by HOLLY R. WYATT, MD

Reader's
digest

New York / Montreal

All images in this book are reprinted courtesy of 3Ball Entertainment, LLC, with the exception of the images on the following pages: 9 Pete Thomas; 17 Stacey Lewis; 19 and 146 Georgeanna Johnson; 23 and 233 Rod Durham; 39 and 182 Elaine Covington; 63 Robert and Raymond Delgado; 70 Jose Flores, Jr.; 87 Mitzi White; 190 Jennifer Callahan; 192 Vanessa Bryan; 208 Joshua Steele

ISBN 978-1-62145-289-8

Library of Congress Cataloging in Publication Data
Names: Roth, JD, (Television producer) author.
Title: The big fat truth : behind-the-scenes secrets to losing weight
and gaining the inner strength to transform your life / by JD Roth.
Description: New York, NY : Trusted Media Brands, Inc., [2016] | Includes index.
Identifiers: LCCN 2015037050| ISBN 9781621452898 (hardback) | ISBN 9781621452904 (epub)
Subjects: LCSH: Weight loss--Psychological aspects. | Nutrition. | Exercise. | BISAC: HEALTH &
FITNESS / Weight Loss. | HEALTH & FITNESS / General. | SELF-HELP / Eating Disorders.
Classification: LCC RM222.2 .R6675 2016 | DDC 613.2--dc23
LC record available at http://lccn.loc.gov/2015037050

We are committed to both the quality of our products and the service we provide to our customers.
We value your comments, so please feel free to contact us.
Reader's Digest Trade Publishing
44 South Broadway
White Plains, NY 10601

For more Reader's Digest products and information, visit our website:
www.rd.com (in the United States)
www.readersdigest.ca (in Canada)

Printed in the United States of America

3 5 7 9 10 8 6 4 2

NOTE TO OUR READERS

The information in this book should not be substituted for, or used to alter, medical therapy without your doctor's advice. For a specific health problem, consult your physician for guidance.

This book is dedicated to all the people who quietly go about changing their lives for the better. They don't make excuses, they don't try fad diets, and they commit to keeping their promises. They tell themselves that they deserve a better life, then they go about making it happen. They are everyday people who were not happy with how they felt about themselves or how they looked in the mirror, and unlike most everyone else in the world, they did something about it.

These people are *you*. I salute your courage in taking on the challenge that lies ahead. And I know you're going to turn what once seemed impossible into your new happy place.

It's always too soon to quit.

Contents

Part III: Now Go Do It!

Foreword

I remember the day I first met JD Roth. It was the final casting week of Season 4 of the TV show *Extreme Weight Loss,* and JD was flying into Denver to inspire the potential new cast members as they prepared for their amazing challenge of losing a life-changing amount of weight in just 365 days. I have to admit I was a little nervous about this meeting and, frankly, very skeptical. Weight loss is my passion—and my specialty. I have spent my career as an academic doctor and researcher studying body weight regulation and designing state-of-the-art interventions to help people lose weight and keep it off. Over the last 20 years, I have worked with Dr. James Hill to develop cutting-edge weight management programs, making the University of Colorado Anschutz Health and Wellness Center the preeminent place in the world to lose weight and transform your life.

While I was enthusiastic about the collaboration between our center and *Extreme Weight Loss,* I was unconvinced that JD, a very lean and fit executive TV producer, could possibly understand what it takes for severely obese, very out-of-shape individuals to achieve permanent weight loss. Obesity is a serious medical disease, and it deserves the very best evidence-based treatment. In the back of my mind I was preparing for what I might have to "undo" after he left to make sure we really got the cast off on the right path for success. To be honest, I was ready for damage control.

To my very relieved and pleasant surprise, JD ended up teaching me a lot about what is really important for effective weight loss. He absolutely does know what it takes to be successful in long-term weight loss. I am happy to report that over the next two years we partnered very productively with JD and *Extreme Weight Loss*. JD's famous casting pep talk is one of my favorites. It is totally aligned with the ways we think about transformative weight loss at our center, and I admit I've borrowed many of his inspirational stories and mantras to motivate some of my toughest patients.

It turns out JD has a true gift, a natural insight into what it really takes to help people lose weight and succeed in life. Perhaps I shouldn't have been shocked by this. As a successful TV producer, he is a student of human nature, of how people react in different situations and how real and deep emotions are usually what rule people's outward behavior. The stories he told on *Extreme Weight Loss* exemplified his ability to find and link that deep emotion to each cast member's goal of losing weight and changing their life . . . the essence of lasting success. He inherently understands that weight loss has to be bigger than a diet and exercise plan. Yes, he is a wildly successful producer, but he is also one hell of a life coach. His tell-it-like-it-is tough love approach is coupled with a true love for every cast member. That makes him a very rare individual who can make people at any size or fitness level believe they can succeed and inspire them do the hard work it takes to win the obesity battle.

I would not blame you if you were also a little skeptical about JD being able to tell you a thing or two about weight loss. But I urge you to give him a chance. JD instinctively knows that the body follows the mind (the seat of emotion), which is absolutely the key for weight loss. Unlike the majority of weight loss books, his book is designed to change your mind-set before you change your diet or your waist size. This book is not about the best diet or exercise plan; there are lots of other books out there that can help you with that. This book is about the power of believing in yourself, the power of deciding you are not going to let the excuses you have used for so long stand in your way, the power to finally go and do it.

The Big Fat Truth will make you uncomfortable, and it should. If you do not cry and sweat a little when you read this book—and feel uneasy and a little excited at the same time—you did not dig deep enough. Being comfortable is keeping you right where you are today: unhappy, unmotivated, and sitting on the sidelines. Being uncomfortable is where the JD magic really starts. JD sees a much bigger and brighter future for you. This book will not only help you see it, too, but it will help you believe you can get there.

So if you are ready to stop playing the blame game, get rid of the victim mentality, and stop looking for a magic bullet for your weight problems . . . if you are ready to be your own hero and do the work as the star of your own TV show, you are absolutely reading the right book.

The power to change your life once and for all is already inside of you. Sprinkle a little JD magic from this book into your personal recipe to find it, believe it, and finally take a BIG step in the direction of your oh-so-POSSIBLE dream.

Believing it is always the first step to seeing it! JD can help you believe.

With much love, light, and gratitude,
Dr. Holly

Holly R. Wyatt, MD
Associate Professor, University of Colorado School of Medicine
Medical Director, University of Colorado
Anschutz Health and Wellness Center
Medical Director, Seasons 4 and 5, *Extreme Weight Loss*
Co-Author, *The State of Slim*

Introduction

Why? Why haven't you lost weight yet? Please tell me you have a reason. It can't just be that you are hungry. No one is *that* hungry.

You're willing to get to the bottom of a carton of ice cream, but are you willing to get to the bottom of why you are overeating? If you're ever going to transform your body, you need to be. So get out a piece of paper and a pencil, and write down four answers to the question above.

I don't even know you, but I can venture to name a few of the things that you might write.

> "I'm crazy busy."
> "I'm stressed."
> "I have the fat gene."
> "I don't like exercise."
> "I can only afford fast food."
> "I'm Latina, Italian, Jewish—eating is part of my
>   culture."
> "I have no willpower."
> "My dad abused me."
> "My whole family died."

Now take your pencil and next to each answer write "EXCUSE!"

> "I'm crazy busy." *EXCUSE!*
> "I'm stressed." *EXCUSE!*

1

"I have the fat gene." *EXCUSE!*
"I don't have time to exercise." *EXCUSE!*
"I can only afford fast food." *EXCUSE!*
"I'm Latina, Italian, Jewish—eating is part of my
   culture." *EXCUSE!*
"I have no willpower." *EXCUSE!*
"My dad abused me." *EXCUSE!*
"My whole family died." *EXCUSE!*

The reasons you listed for not losing weight may all be true statements, but none of them—not even those last two, harsh as it sounds—entitle you to destroy your health. Even when something horrible happens, there comes a point when you have to pick up the pieces and pay attention to your well-being. So stop telling yourself that the reasons you came up with are good ones, because they're not. In fact, I can tell without even seeing them that they suck. They are stopping you from not only wearing a smaller dress or pants size, but from living a quality life.

Imagine, instead, a world where you say to yourself, "I'm tense and angry—I need to go take a boxing class to get rid of the stress" instead of, "I'm tense and angry—I need to eat some cake." Or one where taking a salsa class or studying the language of your heritage replaces blaming the way you eat as respect for your culture. Whether you know it or not, you have the potential to dramatically change your inner dialogue and, with it, your life. And it's not just about losing weight. What I'm talking about is becoming a happier, more vibrant, and more empowered person. Someone who does things they never thought possible.

How do you get to that point? Not with any miracle diet and exercise program. You get there by changing the way you think. It is your mind-set that guides what you put in your mouth and your decision to sit on the couch, pizza in hand, when you should be moving your body. Whether you have 10 pounds or a 100 pounds to lose, **the big fat truth is you are carrying that weight in your head.** I don't mean that you're imagining it, but that your body is only a reflection of what is in your head. You're not fat because you love food. It's your mind-set that's keeping you shopping in the plus-size section. And unless you get to the root of the problem, you'll be shopping there until the day you die (which, let's be honest, if you're very overweight, has the potential to come sooner than you may like). But fix what's going on in your brain and your body will follow.

Here's another critical factor: choosing to believe in yourself. It's that simple. Believe in yourself, and you'll look back at that list of excuses and laugh at how ridiculous they were.

Even if you don't believe in yourself yet, I *already* believe in you. As the man who invented weight-loss TV with shows like *The Biggest Loser, Extreme Weight Loss, Fat Chance,* and *The Revolution,* I have seen so many people—many of them seemingly hopeless cases—transform themselves right before my very eyes that I know you can do it, too. So even though I'm going to say things that may make you flinch, feel hurt, and even piss you off—I do it because these are hard truths you need to hear. But there is a great big payoff. By the time I get done with you, you'll be able to wear a glazed-doughnut necklace (with sprinkles!) around your neck 24 hours a day, and not feel the slightest bit of temptation. I'm going to wake the sleeping beast within you—a beast that is immune to the tastiest of french fries and the chocolatiest of chocolate cakes. Really.

If you've picked up this book, you are probably fat. Maybe you're really fat, or maybe you're not all that fat but you know you've been abusing yourself by living on junk food and sitting on your butt. The people who try out for my shows have these problems in a big way. They usually need two airplane seats to make the trip to our casting calls, then endure sitting on a tiny, unbelievably uncomfortable chair for hours, all because things in their lives are not going well.

My guess is that things are not going well for you either. Your weight and unhealthy living is robbing you of a good life. Maybe you've had years of disappointments, self-doubt, self-loathing, bad relationships, and bad jobs. Even your car may be a disaster. I wouldn't be surprised, either, if you have an overwhelming feeling that you are unworthy of happiness. Love, pleasure, prosperity: They're for other people. That is the mantra that swirls around in your head. And you couldn't be more wrong. You deserve everything that everyone else has. Your life has the potential to be 100 percent better—even if from where you're sitting right now, dramatic changes seem overwhelming. They're not. Don't use that as an excuse to not do what you know you need to do. Instead, take action; take control.

The rewards of a successful weight-loss journey far exceed simply looking better. Looking good is great; we all want to look good. But you have the opportunity to change your life in a much more profound way—just like so many of the participants in our weight-loss shows have. As they shed weight, they get off serious medications, they go places, and they do things that they had never done before or had been avoiding for years. Most significantly, they get their lives back by resolving the issues that made them fat in the first place. As the person who has final say on who will appear on the shows, and the behind-the-scenes guy in charge of inspiring, persuading, and prodding (and okay, sometimes yelling at) contestants to stay committed to change, I have seen people overcome the most horrific obstacles to reshape their bodies and their lives. And if they can do it, so can you.

This book is here to help. It's not a diet book. Yes, I sprinkle some eating and exercise advice throughout, but I will not be giving you a food plan or any of the other typical advice you find in a diet book. (I will, however, give you the typical disclaimer you'll get in a diet book, which is that you should always consult with your doctor before trying any sort of weight loss plan, especially if you have any chronic health issues.) I don't even believe in diets—the kind you go on, then go off later. What I'm offering you instead is something much more critical: strategies for changing your perspective, your attitude, your *whole* approach to weight loss. Discovering the *real* reasons those pounds have piled on can be painful, it can create anxiety, and it can take time to heal. But life without introspection can be even darker.

And life without introspection doesn't bode well for weight loss. That's something on which I've staked my career. When my partner, Todd, and I pitched our first reality show to the networks, we were told to go away and come back with doctors and other weight-loss experts who would confirm that we could get people to safely lose dramatic amounts of weight on a weekly basis. After all, what did we know? We were just television producers. We called every well-known weight-loss center in the country and talked to every specialist we could find, and *none* of them believed we could do it. Zero. "People can't lose more than one to two pounds a week," we were told again and again. At that rate, it would take at least a year to get weight off our show's contestants, and that wasn't going to fly on TV. "If your cast loses only one to two pounds a week, you'll be off the air in a week," said one of the network execs.

Somehow, we got the go-ahead from NBC to do it our way. The night before the first official weigh-in—the moment when the cast members get on the scale and learn how well they've done that week—we secretly weighed the contestants. If it was going to be bad, we wanted to know ahead of time. Only we could see the numbers on the scale (a special system we created so we could build the drama) so the guy's reaction when he got on the scale for the cameras the next day would be real.

I wish I had our own reaction on tape: The cast member had lost *16 pounds in less than a week*. Not one or two pounds, as every medical expert has told us to expect, but *16*. Todd and I couldn't believe our eyes. We made him get on and off the scale three more times just to make sure it was right. The two of us were jumping for joy. That week, everyone in the cast lost weight in the double digits. Collectively, they went on to lose 768 pounds over the 16-week season. Suddenly, all those weight-loss experts who had turned us down earlier went from thinking we were crazy and irresponsible to asking us for our data so they could use it in their own research. So what was it? The secret ingredient that helped us annihilate what the experts told us was impossible?

What I believe we—and all the people who've appeared on our shows—have proven is that addressing your mental and emotional blocks is the secret to sustained weight loss. Nobody was dealing with people's heads and hearts; they were dealing with science (calories in, calories out, and all that stuff). But science can only get you so far. We discovered that *love* was the secret ingredient needed to bake the perfect weight-loss cake. We really believe in our cast members, and we truly love them. They can see it in our eyes. Throughout this book, you'll hear me say how important it is to have supportive people around you. That's not just psychology 101—we have thousands of TV episodes to prove it.

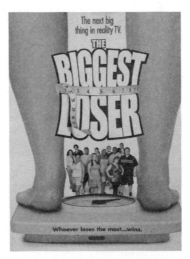

Poster for the first season of
The Biggest Loser.

* * * * *

Everyone has different underlying reasons for being overweight, but one thing that everyone shares is responsibility. Yes, you are to blame for the fat body you're in. I'm not saying there aren't other guilty parties: the fast-food makers, taunting you with images of double-decker, cheese-soaked, bacon-wrapped burgers at dirt-cheap prices. Places that serve not glasses of soda, but buckets. Supermarkets full of microwaveable meals as quick and easy as they are caloric-laden. Cookies, ice cream, candy, fattening coffee drinks that taste so-o-o-o-o good. Food scientists have become experts at mixing up just the right amount of salt and sugar needed to trigger the brain chemicals that send you into ecstasy. They know what they're doing just as surely as the tobacco companies and corner drug dealers know how to ensure repeat business: Studies have shown that sugar and fat can cause cravings as potent as those caused by cocaine and nicotine.

So, yeah, we're all up against it. With temptation raining down all around, it's not for nothing that close to 70 percent of American adults are fat. You heard me, 70 percent! Yet when it comes down to it, the buck must stop with the person who's lifting the fork up to your mouth: YOU! You are to blame for making choices that got you to this point in your life. One day, you decided to stop caring about your health and well-being—maybe your relationships, your job, and your feelings, too—and started to settle for less in every area of your life. Then, once you gave in to accepting less . . . well, eating became even easier.

Maybe you're asking yourself, why should I take weight-loss advice from a TV guy? True, I am a TV guy, but first and foremost, I'm a problem-solving guy, and always have been. I was the kid in school who everyone came to with their problems, including my twin sister. She's now a pediatrician, but when she was struggling in medical school, I spent a lot of time countering her glass-half-empty temperament with my glass-half-full coaching. Back before email and texting (when you actually had to write letters by hand), I sent her cards and letters encouraging her to hang in there—to live in the solution, not in the problem. I know sometimes I sound like a fortune cookie, but the things I believe in work. I had no idea that she kept every card and letter I ever wrote to her until twenty years later, when I turned forty, she bound them all up into a book and gave them back to me as a gesture of thanks. I love her for it, and for the effort she made to go from negative to positive thinking. She is now a very successful doctor because of that effort.

This is all by way of saying that I love nothing more than seeing people learn to fight for their dreams, then go on to achieve them like my twin sister did. I live for it. And my natural inclination to jump in and help people with their problems has served me well in my role as a producer. Of course, it's the role of all the shows' technicians—the trainers, the nutritionists, the doctors, and others—to guide the show contestants through the day-to-day rigors of weight loss, and they do an amazing job. You can see that on-screen.

However, when the cameras are off, I'm often the one who swoops in to stop the contestants from zipping up their suitcases and quitting, then getting them fired up enough to master the Herculean tasks in front of them—because I know they can do it! From the day they walk in the door to try out for the show to the day they walk out, I'm the guy on a mission to lift them up when their motivation is flagging and talk them down when their willpower is lagging. I give them pep talks. I call them. I text them. I get in their faces. For that reason, I'm the guy whose picture they tape onto their elliptical trainers and angrily scream at at night—then hug the next morning because they're so proud of what they've accomplished. I'm the guy who holds them when they cry and the one who tells them they need to get back on the treadmill even though they're swearing they can't take another step. I'm the tough-love dad who challenges them to do more than they have ever done before. After they leave the show, I still keep in touch and mentor many of them as they continue to forge new lives for themselves. One former cast member, Pete, sends me a picture of himself every year on the anniversary of his final weigh-in. He is still as lean as the day he left the show more than 10 years ago.

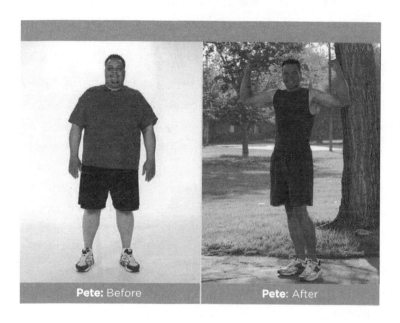

Pete: Before **Pete:** After

The Biggest Loser, Extreme Weight Loss (originally called *Extreme Makeover: Weight Loss Edition*), and the other transformational shows I've developed over the last 12 years have allowed me to meet some of the most amazing people. It's my job to inspire them, but they inspire *me*. Working on the shows has also given me a bird's-eye view of the difficulties overweight people contend with every day—although not for the first time. Everyone in my family, immediate and extended, except me, has struggled with their weight at one time or another.

Despite what I do for a living, many of my family members have a very different outlook on food, nutrition, and exercise than mine. Technically, my twin, the pediatrician, knows there's a difference between having a sugary cereal versus a flaxseed waffle for breakfast—she studied nutritional biochemistry at Cornell and finished in the top of her class! But when she feeds her daughters, I see in her what I see in thousands of busy working moms: Sometimes, it's just easier to go for the box of cereal when you have a kid to get to school and patients to care for. (Recently, she has converted to a plant-based lifestyle, and I am so happy!)

My younger sister has struggled with her weight since she was a teenager, and I know her quality of life could be so much better if she dropped some pounds and made it a priority to set an example of living healthfully for her kids. But once again, as an accomplished lawyer and single mom of fraternal twins, she constantly sacrifices herself for the sake of her busy schedule and mom duties.

My mom, for her part, went to Weight Watchers every Monday for almost 25 years ("Mom," I tell her, "it's not working . . .") and has an aversion to exercise. When I was growing up, a hike for my mom was trekking through Bloomingdale's, and that's still pretty much how things stand today. Her theory is that you're only allowed so many heartbeats in your life and that working out uses them up too quickly. (I wish I was kidding!)

My dad has an even crazier story. He was the COO of a very large hospital on the East Coast and is one of the smartest businessmen I know. Forget the fact that he's in a medical environment every day; he thinks that eating 15 pieces of bacon for breakfast and three sausage sandwiches, hold the bread, for lunch, is a diet ("because Dr. Atkins said so"). One day, he walked into a meeting at the hospital and felt a pain in his chest. He took out his key card, quietly let himself into the cardiac unit, and proceeded to have a heart attack. Within 15 minutes, they had a stent in his heart. How lucky is that? If he'd been home, he probably wouldn't have made it. So after this traumatic episode, I'm thinking, *This is it, now he's going to change, finally listen to his son, and lose the weight that probably contributed to sending him into the cardiac unit.*

"Hey, Dad," I say, "you're going to change your life now, right? Eat better, exercise?"

"Naw," he tells me. "At 69 years old, these things happen." The following Tuesday after the heart attack, he was at a local steakhouse finishing off a New York strip with a glass of red wine.

These things happen? You mean heart attacks? Come on! These things don't *have* to happen if you use all that brainpower toward good! They're my family, and I love them—but I knew from a young age that I didn't think like them. And for what it's worth, they think I am a little crazy in the opposite direction. Why do I exercise so much? What do I have against eating meat? They may be right; I can go to extremes. But healthy extremes. An error on my side does not give you a heart attack.

Plus, from an early age, I seemed to have a different constitution. I'd go out to play basketball and come back seven hours later. I couldn't sit still. But it wasn't always easy to buck the family way of life. Growing up, every night at eight o'clock, there was a race to the freezer to pull out the Breyer's chocolate-chip ice cream. (My mouth waters just writing it down!) We each got a coffee cup and were allowed to mash as much ice cream as possible into its interior. By the time I got done with mine, it took two hands to lift it off the counter. The memories of that ritual give me a lot of happiness, but at almost 50 years old, if I was still doing that I would be in the same category as 70 percent of America . . . overweight and wondering how it happened!

Most days, my mom packed us kosher salami sandwiches, potato chips, and a vanilla creme Dunkin' Donut for lunch. (I loved it! And it came with a note about how much she loved us.) But, in those days, every other family was doing the same thing. I didn't even know there was another way to eat. About all we knew of vegetables was corn on the cob and maybe some tomatoes in the summer. (It was Jersey! You had to have tomatoes. We were famous for our tomatoes!) The Jersey culture went something like this: If you were happy, "Let's go get a cheesesteak." If you lost a game, "Let's go get a cheesesteak." Cheesesteaks solved every problem. They were used for both celebration and when cheering up was necessary. My picture still hangs in the most famous cheesesteak house in the United States, Jim's Steaks on South Street in Philly. I can smell the grilled onions as I write this!

These days, I am so not that guy (and my kids are so not those kids). I made a conscious effort not to go down that path, especially when I discovered how great it felt to be fit and eat healthfully. I also happened to marry someone who is committed to feeding us healthfully. It's my wife's passion; therefore, it is my passion, too. If her passion was ice cream and fresh pastries that would also be hard to avoid. You are who you hang out with when it comes to food. Family pressures are especially hard to shake, and that's something I'll deal with at length in this book. Families don't like outliers; if they're fat, they want you to be fat, too. If they're not fat and you are, it can be just as bad. Nothing can make your rebellious fingers dial pizza delivery quicker than parents who criticize your weight. We'll talk about that challenge, too.

* * * * *

I know that you know how to lose weight. Eat less, move more—it's not exactly rocket science. In fact, it's simple; most problem solving is. I'll give you an example. A few years ago, my oldest son, Cooper, came home from school crying.

"I've got a book report due in the morning! I forgot about it! I haven't started it. What am I going to do?!" He was in a complete panic, tears streaming down his face.

"Okay, stop," I said. "What's step number one?"

"Identify the problem." (As you can see, we've been down this road before—he knows the drill.)

"Well, what's the problem?"

"I've got a book report that's due tomorrow, and I haven't even read the book."

"Okay, great, what's step number two?"

"Make a list," he says.

And he goes on to make the list: read the book, do a drawing, write an outline, then write the report.

"Great. What's step number three?"

He's stopped crying now, and he's completely calm. He looks down and says, "I know what step number three is Dad."

"Well, what is it?"

"Go do it." He was now in control of what a few minutes ago had seemed like an impossible situation.

Cooper started working on his report at about 3:00 p.m. He came down about four hours later, and said he was done. I asked him if he gave it his best.

"Dad, I am going to get an A," he said.

"That is not what I asked you," I replied. "Did you give that report your best work?"

"No, I did not do my best."

I told Cooper to go back upstairs and give me his best. He did, and *then* he was right. He did get an A. In fact, it was one of the best papers he ever wrote.

This three-step solution solves just about any problem. My son is learning how to use it at an early age, but if you've never had much practice reaching step three, it can be difficult to change. Most people in life never get to step three, especially where weight loss is concerned. So what I'm saying is that it doesn't matter if eating less and moving more is a simple formula for transforming the body, *if you don't do it*. (And by "do it," I mean do it for a lifetime.) You can know all the diet tricks and best ways to burn fat in the gym—in fact, you probably already do—but, of course, if you're not putting them to use, the problem will not be solved. Replace the fat thoughts in your head with the mantra, "Do it." Say it over and over to yourself! Every day, in every situation. Talking about your dreams of being a thin, fit person is fun . . . but actually being a thin, fit person is even more fun! So stop talking about it. Instead, "do it!"

One of the big goals of this book is to make a believer of you, to fire you up, and to help you realize that you actually have a deep well of strength and willpower inside you, just waiting to be tapped. But even more important, I want to help you truthfully answer the question, *Why aren't I just doing it? What is stopping me from doing the work it takes to give myself a better life? Why don't I think I deserve it?*

I make every participant on our shows ask themselves these questions. One of them was Stacey, a 42-year-old woman, who tried out for *The Revolution*, a daytime weight-loss show I produced a few years back. (*The Revolution*, in case you missed it, was a daily show on ABC daytime where all the cast members were women. We not only helped them lose weight, we helped them make over their homes and personal style. Ty Pennington and Tim Gunn were hosts.) It was casting's make-or-break moment, and Stacey was being given a final chance to convince us that we should put her on TV. So in she came to the last-chance room, taking a seat in one of those small chairs.

"Stacey," I asked her, "tell us how you got to this point in your life."

"I have been married to a fantastic man for 20 years," she began, "I have three kids, and I love food."

"No, you don't," I said.

She laughed nervously. "Yes, I do. I love the taste in my mouth, I love to cook food; I love everything about food."

"Your weight has nothing to do with food," I told her. This is usually the moment where people start looking at me sideways, thinking I am trying to trick them. I am actually trying to get them to honestly look inward; that can be very hard.

"Well, of course it does. How do you think I got to over 300 pounds? By eating broccoli?" She let out a huge infectious laugh that got the whole room blessing it with an "Amen."

‖‖

Something Lost, Something Gained

JD,

There are people in world who do a lot of dreaming and talking. Yet, at the end of the day they do not produce results (I used to be one of them). So-o-o-o-o-o-o-o-o many wonderful things have happened to me during this journey: I am liberated from my past demons; I have lost more than 50 pounds (and counting); and I am confidence personified. Yet, the thing that has left the greatest impression for me is that I have the honor to see what truly can happen when a person not only dreams but puts calculated action behind their desires.

—Stacey, *The Revolution* cast member, via email

I was honest with her. "Look, Stacey, you're a nice, warm person, but I don't see you going to a *real* deep emotional place. I need you to tell me something that happened to you that you haven't even told your husband or mother about. If you really want to have us choose you and help you change your life, you have to reveal something no one has ever heard before. Something so scary to you that you have put it in a place so deep and hidden from view that just thinking about it makes you want to reach for a sheet cake and demolish it in one sitting."

And just like that, in a matter of seconds, Stacey's deepest, darkest secret—something that she had held onto for more than 30 years—came pouring out as if it happened yesterday. And once the silence was broken, the pain came rushing out faster then all the lines of BS about how much she loved food.

Stacey admitted, right there in that chair, in front of ten people she barely knew, that as a young girl she was sexually abused. She'd never told her husband or her mother. She kept this secret, living in her own private hell and using food to shove those feelings down as far as they would go. But, of course, there are not enough cookies in the world, not enough BBQ ribs on this planet, to make that kind of devastation and fear go away. The room went silent. Stacey was sobbing uncontrollably. All I wanted to do was hug her but I held back, and after what felt like an hour (though was probably more like 30 seconds) of stillness and listening to her cries of rage, I said in a whisper, "You know what you need to do, right?"

She said nothing. I went on. "You need to go home tonight and tell your husband everything." The whole room let out a gasp, as if I had just used a racial epithet.

Looking fear in the face and doing what frightens you anyway is *living*. The very thing that scares you the most might also surprise you the most. I told Stacey that if she wanted to get on the show, she would need to confront the very thing that terrified her most. Telling her husband that she was abused as a child was the start of her journey. **The root of transformation is desire.** Without the desire to follow through and act on this scary suggestion, the opportunity could vanish in an instant. This was not about TV anymore. It was about something much bigger. It was about healing. No matter what happened from that moment on, her life *had* to get better simply because she'd no longer be carrying that burden around. The fat on Stacey's body was not the end product of 10,000 Oreo cookies and 5,000 Big Macs; it was the weight of evil that had been tormenting her for 30 years.

Of course, food was involved. How can you be married to someone you love for more than 20 years and have a secret that big, that personal, and still carry on as if it never happened? I'll tell you how. You eat lots and lots and lots of food. Then one day, you wake up 300 pounds and three kids later, and you realize that your shame and pain have now been transferred to them, that they're starting to show signs of obesity and anxiety, too. And it hurts even more.

So you eat even more. Until one day, you don't. One day, you tell the truth, and you start the healing. Every tear you cry lightens you by one pound and puts you one step closer to conquering what's been standing in your way. You start to win. You start to take control of a life that has been out of control for too long.

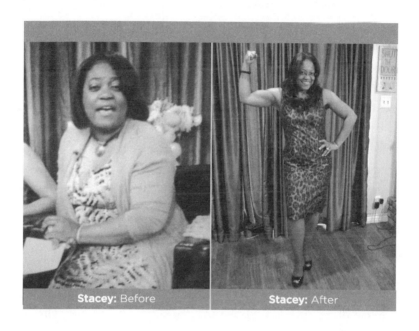

Stacey: Before   Stacey: After

The day after Stacey had made her big confession, she came back for a final audition. When I saw her, she practically tackled me, hugging me as she cried. I held her for a few moments, then she told me something amazing.

"Wha . . . What happened?" I asked her, feeling a little nervous about the outcome.

When Stacey went home the night before, she couldn't sleep. Late in the evening, she told her husband her secret. He began crying, and she feared the worst. Maybe he wouldn't understand. Maybe he'd think she was damaged goods and walk away from the marriage. In fact, it was the opposite; he understood too well. Unbelievably, he revealed that the same thing had happened to him as a child. They both had been holding onto a terrible secret all throughout their marriage—sleeping in the same bed for 20 years, having the same nightmare, only to wake up and fake it for another day. They kept secrets from each other out of love, but it hurt both of them in the long term. The willingness to see something in someone's eyes and not ask questions was probably one of the very things that attracted them to each other. It bonded them in some sort of twisted empathy that allowed the secret to live on but only in silence. It also allowed them to love each other unconditionally. Beautiful and sad at the same time.

Stacey made it onto the show, and if you see her today, she looks amazing. She said her marriage started over that night, and they have never been happier.

Stacey's story is very, very dramatic—a lot of the people who participate in our shows have dramatic stories. That's TV. But we have also had people on our shows whose narratives are so common that I'm sure thousands of readers share them. If you can't see yourself in a story like Stacey's, you may be able to relate to Georgeanna's.

When Georgeanna tried out for *Extreme Weight Loss*, she didn't think she'd make it on the show—there had been no abuse or other craziness in her life. And that's exactly why we wanted her. Georgeanna weighed in at 315 pounds when she started. A former gymnast and cheerleader, she became pregnant during college, dropped out, got married, and spent the next 23 years devoting herself to her husband and two daughters (while holding down a job, too). The first few years were stressful; money was tight and Georgeanna didn't really know how to feed a family properly. But she was also intent on proving that, despite having gotten off to an unplanned start, she could be a great mom. "I just lost focus on who I was," she said. In the end, Georgeanna proved she had a great "family plan"; she just didn't have a great "me plan."

Family life got pretty crazy. Running from one daughter's volleyball game to another, eating out all the time, and a general lack of healthy habits all conspired to make her fat. Georgeanna succeeded at being a great mom and failed at taking care of herself. It was when her kids went off to college that she finally realized she didn't have a "me plan." Yet, when she finally committed to turning things around, she lost 150 pounds. Hear that? *One hundred fifty pounds*. Say it out loud because it seems impossible. But what I'm trying to get across is that the impossible *is* possible. Get your head and heart into it, and the weight will come off.

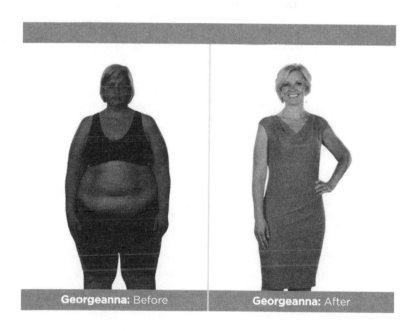

Georgeanna: Before   Georgeanna: After

Georgeanna's biggest problem was that she got caught in a parenting rut. Ask yourself where in your life are you stuck? And then let me help you get un-stuck. In a bad marriage, a job you hate, still living at home, not happy with your social life? Forgive yourself for being in the situation you are in, then start living in the solution. Actively change. Keep taking steps forward to improve your life. I know you are saying right now, "Easy for him to say." It is never easy for anyone, including me, but people who work toward attaining success in every area of their lives don't make excuses; instead, they look at obstacles as inspiration to make progress. Nobody gets it right all the time, but people who succeed keep trying until they get the desired outcome.

* * * * *

The cast members on our shows have a lot of help: trainers to put them through their paces, cooks to make them healthy food, nutritionists to give them diet tricks, me to inspire and push them, and the cameras as an incentive to avoid failure (no one wants to crash and burn in front of millions of viewers). But you'd be wrong to think that you can't do the same thing without all these trappings. First of all, there is no end to weight-loss resources out there, and I'll give you some suggestions in the Resources section to help you find them. Believe me when I tell you that the main reason our contestants shed pounds and keep them off is because they deal with their issues and shift their attitudes about what they're capable of. **The big fat truth is that the game is in your head!** Fix your head, and you'll lose the fat. That's something anyone can do anywhere, anytime—and it's hands-down the most important part of the journey. Actually it *is* the journey. No piece of exercise equipment you have to buy on QVC at 1:00 a.m. No $50-a-day super-fantastic cleanse. Just working an organ/muscle you already have. It's called your brain. Once you change your mind-set and start saying, "I can" instead of "I can't," the pounds just roll off. I've seen it time and time again. Remember: to make something happen, you have to put it out there in the universe. Seems silly to even write this, but I deeply know this to be true on every level of life, not just weight loss.

That reminds me of a story I heard about the actor Jim Carrey. When he first moved to L.A. to become a star, he was poor and practically living out of his car. He wanted to be a star more than anything, so he pulled out his checkbook (even though his bank account was empty) and wrote a check to himself for $10,000,000. For those of you having trouble getting past all those zeros, that's ten million dollars! Then he told himself that one day he was going to deposit that check. He put it in his wallet, and then let that check drive his passion to succeed. Every time he went into his wallet to pull out the few lousy bucks he did have, he saw that check. Every time he reached in to grab his credit card, he saw that check. It was a constant reminder that he had to become famous so he could one day cash that check. Guess what? Years later, he was in a position to cash that check many times over. It was a brain game all along, and it paid off. So what will be your inspiration? What will you put in your wallet to motivate you to live a full, healthy life? You need to make emotional deposits so when it comes time to make a withdrawal, you are secure in yourself, and have what you want out of life.

Throughout the years, people have criticized our production company, saying we exploit fat people for financial gain. It started before the first episode of *The Biggest Loser* even aired. In 2004, the night before our premiere, before the whole genre of weight-loss TV had even hatched, I was asked to come on *Entertainment Tonight* to counter claims by the National Association to Advance Fat Acceptance. Never mind that they hadn't seen a frame of the show; they knew I was a horrible person. On the show, I sat next to two 400-plus pound women, who argued that there are plenty of overweight people that are happy. Why were we trying to say that all overweight people were miserable? It was their gotcha moment. What did I think of that? When the camera cut to me (on a severe close-up, perhaps meant to see me sweat), I looked right into the lens and calmly said, "I'm looking for the ones that are unhappy, and I think there's a lot of them." Conversation over.

If you're a stable, happy, loving, confident person and your body isn't perfect, it doesn't really matter. But I think you also have to ask yourself if you are healthy. Consider that according to the 2009 European Prospective Investigation Into Cancer and Nutrition-Potsdam (EPIC) study, not smoking, exercising 3.5 hours a week, eating a healthy diet, and maintaining a healthy weight prevented 93 percent of diabetes, 81 percent of heart attacks, 50 percent of strokes, and 36 percent of all cancers in a group of 23,000 people. Doesn't that make changing your body and how your treat it, worth it?

I'd ask you, too, are you using food to push down issues you should be dealing with? Are you living the best life you can live? Don't you want to live to see your kids have kids? Do you want to live a healthier lifestyle? Are there things you can't do because of your size?

One contestant, Rod, told me that one of the most humiliating moments of his life was when a flight attendant asked him (loudly) if he needed a seat-belt extender. And there were other mortifying accommodations he had had to make because of his weight. He'd always try to get to a restaurant before his friends so he could look at the chairs to see if they'd hold his weight (booths were out of the question—he couldn't fit in them).

Granted, these are not the problems of every overweight person, but even if it's just having everyone watch you to see what the fat person's going to eat, life can be difficult when you're packing extra pounds. And it's a vicious cycle. As soon as you feel the shame and embarrassment of people looking at you, you're done. Next up is feeling that you are less then everyone else, then accepting less because you think that's all you deserve. Toward the end of his year with us, by the way, Rod sent me a triumphant email with the photos on the following page attached that read, "I asked for the extension belt from one flight attendant (as it had been my norm). The other one remarked, 'He doesn't need one, does he?' She was right."

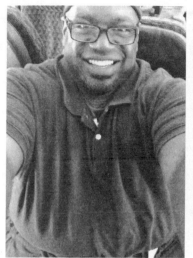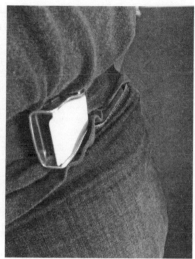

Rod with his seat belt buckled—no extension necessary!

If you've picked up this book, I'm probably preaching to the choir; you are undoubtedly not content with your body, whether it's for health reasons, inconvenience, because you don't think you look good, or all of the above. Nothing wrong with that—though keep in mind that losing weight won't necessarily make you happy. However, getting happy *will* make you lose weight. The two go hand in hand.

Remember the three-pronged principle I told you I drill into my kids? 1) Identify the problem; 2) Make a list of things you need to do; 3) Go do them. That's going to be your assignment, too. This book is divided into three parts, one for each of those principles, plus 30 days' worth of ideas to give you a jump-start. All the chapters are short (I don't want you to feel like you're reading *War and Peace*) and designed to help you come away with insight into your own psyche. Another part of my plan is to give you as much of a reality-weight-loss-show experience as possible. I want you to have the pixie dust that I sprinkle on the participants—and you can, just by reading this book. You may not be on one of our shows, but you can use some of the same tools our cast members do to help them frame their stories and figure out what needs to change. I'll take you through some of the casting process, which will help open up the doors of discovery and begin your transformation.

I want to become your own Miyagi, the character in *The Karate Kid* that teaches his student the right moves by having him practice washing a car (wax on, wax off). That is to say I may ask you to do some things that make you think I am wasting your time. I am not. Trust me, the way I'm going to lead you down the road of change has been proven time and time again. So if I ask you to do something, and you think, "Oh, I can just skip that part," you are once again making excuses for why you can't lose weight.

In the last section of this book, you'll find a 30-day plan full of eating, exercise, and motivational ideas to help you initiate change. Thirty isn't a magic number, but having a month-long "to do" list can help you start the wheels turning. That's important because I don't want you to just contemplate the ideas you'll read about here, I want you to *implement* the ideas immediately. Let the 30-day plan be your guide.

How We Cast Reality Weight-Loss Shows

How do you get a golden ticket? That's what the thousands of people who try out for our weight-loss shows want to know. In truth, no one, two, or even three things automatically qualify you for a spot, and casting differs from show to show. The casting process for *The Biggest Loser* and *Extreme Weight Loss,* though, gives a good picture of what goes through our heads as we try to find the people who will keep television viewers glued to their seats each season.

It goes without saying that you must be considerably overweight to be on one of these shows. But will you be able to lose the weight as millions of viewers watch? That's the first question we ask ourselves anytime we're considering bringing someone into the show's fold. Despite all the trainers and nutritionists and the perfect little bubble they live in for a time (this is called Boot Camp, three months at a health-and-wellness center away from family and friends), the *Extreme Weight Loss* cast must work *very* hard. You have to not just want to change your body, but be willing to tough out all the exertion, dietary changes, and emotional upheavals that make weight loss happen.

As we narrow the group of potential cast members down from thousands of hopefuls, we give the finalists medical tests, and have them fill out a 600-question psych test, triple the number of questions on the California Bar Exam. Yeah, there's a lot of paperwork. (Cast members ultimately asked to join the show are presented with a contract that's about 150 pages!) Those who make the cut spend two weeks with us at the health-and-wellness center where we see how well they do making it to the gym and giving up pizza. Then we monitor them for another month once we send them home, sometimes even keeping an eye on what they're doing when they think we're not looking. Yes, we send spies to monitor if they get to the gym on time, late, or early. We even look at their treadmill times. If you made a promise to run for 60 minutes and got off at 58 minutes, you are not ready to transform. These are key indicators for success. So, if you are not really invested in the process, you get left on the side of the road. We can't fill out the forms for you, and we can't pedal your legs on the bike for you. All we can do is show you the road, and promise to be there to hold your hand.

Every year, our casting process has gotten longer and more complex, but it's paid off: Out of 55 contestants on *Extreme Weight Loss*, we've only had two people drop out—that's 53 people who changed their lives for the better. And with well over a thousand contestants on *The Biggest Loser*, the numbers are even more impressive. (But seeing the episodes where two people took failure as an option was instructive. I think many viewers could see themselves in those people and identify with the choices they made.) One of the most amazing things I've learned while watching these transformations is that success is addictive. At the very start of filming, I can honestly say that we want the cast members to lose weight more than even they do themselves. Some of them, believe it or not, considering all they go through to get on the show, are still a little on the fence. But by the end, they are ravenous for success.

I know this is going to happen for you, too. Once you get a taste of victory, you'll want more. It's exactly like that first bite of the three-layer devil's food cake you love—it just makes you want more. Only this is a healthy addiction. And transformation is so much sweeter than that bite of devil's food cake!

Another important part of this book is the stories I tell about the cast members who have appeared on my shows—and who provide the evidence that my method works. Throughout these pages, you will hear from many of the people who've had success (as well as their ups and downs) with weight loss. They gained incredible knowledge while going through the process and have words of wisdom to offer. I still keep in touch with many former cast members, and you'll see excerpts from their emails, posts, and texts scattered throughout the book, giving you an idea of their progress and the battles they still fight every day. You'll also read success stories that are going to make you want to dump the contents of your refrigerator and jump up and run five miles. They're that inspiring.

I'm going to tell you truths that you may not want to hear, but will be glad you did. Most of all, I'm going to give you hope. Hope has lead many men for thousands of years into battle, hope is the basis for every religion on the planet, and hope even elected the president of the United States! Hope is a key ingredient in the game of change, but hope has to have action behind it. Hoping you will get thin, and not doing anything about it will never get you closer to your goals. But you can do this! The job ahead of you isn't for the faint of heart; it's not for the weak (but don't worry if you feel weak now, this book is going to show you how strong you really are). Losing weight for good is entirely within your realm of possibility. Starting now, your life will be divided into *before* you became the master of your fate and *after* you took the reins.

Are you all in? Then bring it!

PART I

IDENTIFY THE PROBLEM

CHAPTER 1

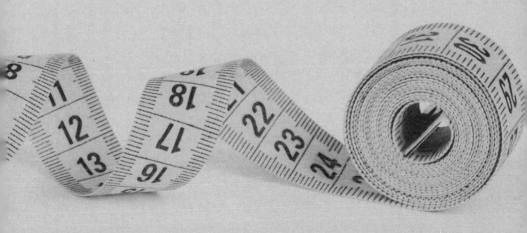

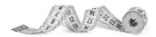

Are You Ready to Lose Weight? No, I Mean Really, Truly Ready?

What person buying a book on weight loss isn't ready to lose weight? It sounds like an idiotic question. But if you're going to identify why you're still fat and having to buy this book in the first place, you have to pinpoint what went wrong in the past. Maybe you just weren't ready. The question is: Are you ready now?

Here's one way to know for sure. Ask yourself if you're willing to give up on the idea of a quick fix. You know what I'm talking about. The magic workout that delivers thin thighs in three days. The cleanse that guarantees to slim you down in just a week. Five-minute-a-day exercise routines. Soup-only diets. Ab-sculpting gadgets that you can own in three easy payments. If you're ready to say no to all these gimmicks, then yes, you're moving in the right direction.

Quick-fix gimmicks make me crazy. The promises made in many diet books, on infomercials, and on magazine covers work all right—they work to make billions of dollars for the people that hawk them. They get fat wallets, and you're still fat! If any one of those "remedies" actually did the job, there'd never be another one invented. We could all go home. Just like if all it took was five minutes a day to get abs like the guy on TV pushing some workout contraption, we'd all be dating supermodels. But it just isn't true. None of it. You have a better chance of winning the lottery than getting thin with these empty promises.

||||||||||||||||||||||||||||||||||||||||||||||||||||||||||||||||||||||||||||||

The Secret to Weight Loss? There Is No Secret

I'm pretty chummy with the security guard at my local bank. I'd just left the bank and our conversation went a little something like this:

Guard: Hey . . . haven't seen you in a while, how are you?

Me: Great, how are you?

Guard (staring at me with his mouth open): Can I ask you something?

Me: Sure, what's up?

Guard: Wow . . . are you losing weight?

Me: Aww . . . yes, I am trying.

Guard: What's the secret?

Me (whispering): Eating healthy and exercising.

Guard: No . . . come on, tell me. How are you losing weight?

Me: I'm serious.

Guard: Whatever.

Hahhhhha-a-a-a. Wow! I wish people knew . . . there's no big secret, and if I can do it, they can do it!

—Jamilla, posted on *The Revolution* Facebook page

Anyone who falls for these gimmicks (and I'm betting you've tried your share of them in the past) wants to believe that there's an easy way to get fit and thin so they don't have do the work. You're fooling yourself if you think the girl in the seven-minutes-to-a-better-butt workout video looks the way she looks because she used that routine a few times a week. Her job is to be fit and thin and, guaranteed, she works at it *hours* not minutes, and not just a few times a week, but *every day*. No doubt, too, she's living on a diet of steamed broccoli and grilled chicken. She might have even given up drinking any liquids for 24 hours before the shoot to make herself look even leaner in front of the camera, and then painted herself the perfect even medium brown tan (remember, I'm in the TV business. I know how they do this stuff!). The fact that millions of people buy into these pipe dreams only proves P. T. Barnum's famous line: "There's a sucker born every minute."

So first things first. Don't be a sucker one second longer. Stop thinking that magician David Blaine is going to wave his magic wand over your belly and make it disappear. If you're serious about losing weight, you'll stop taking the path of least resistance, and get to work! What I'm asking you to do hurts (sometimes literally). Accept the fact that there's no easy way out, and the next time that you'll find yourself pulling out your credit card at midnight to make three easy payments for some pie-in-the-sky gadget will be . . . never!

What are some other signs that you're ready to take on the challenging process of weight loss? One is that you're not just paying lip service to all that you're going to do to make it happen; you actually have a plan. I hear people say they're pumped up and ready to go all the time. Many of them have a determined look and a fire in their eyes that's pretty convincing, too. They'll give me their "Sunday Sermon," a spiel about how committed they are with a laundry list of how they're going to make good on their promises. "I'm going to wake up every day at 4:00 a.m. and exercise!" they'll say. "I'm going to throw everything in my refrigerator and cupboards in the trash!" And yet, these are often the same people who, during casting finals, order steak and fries from room service (did they think we wouldn't find out?). My point is, it's easy to talk a big game, but harder to actually do what you say you will.

It may sound like I'm trying to scare you off. I'm not. I'm just all about being realistic. It's easy to get excited about the prospect of losing weight, but when it comes to doing the actual losing? That's hard. So before you jump in, ensure that this time things really *are* going to be different by doing a little more introspection. Here are five more questions to ask yourself.

1. Are you prepared to make *all* of the lifestyle changes necessary to get you to your end goal?

Every time we put out a casting call for one of our weight-loss shows, thousands of people line up. Who eventually makes the cut depends on a lot of factors, but I can tell you that we always choose people who are absolutely, 100 percent all in. (Or at least they seem to be—I won't say that we've never made a mistake.) These are people so determined to change their lives that they are willing to do whatever we ask of them, no matter how crazy or difficult. And we have had them do some crazy things. One year, we had contestants participate in a competition that involved pulling a burro uphill for 11 miles. It's called the Western Pack Burro Association race and you have to love the motto: "Celebrating 64 years of hauling ass." That race is a fairly extreme test of physical stamina (and of how well you can control a burro, which is not a piece of cake). The craziest thing we ask of contestants, though, is their participation in the one-day 7,000-calorie-burn challenge, an insane undertaking that I'll tell you more about in Chapter 17. Go beyond what you think you can achieve, and the rest is easy.

The lengths people will go to when they're committed continually impresses me. However, the feats that impress me the most require not physical, but emotional stamina. On *The Biggest Loser* and *Extreme Weight Loss*, the cast begins their year with an intensive Boot Camp that requires them to leave behind their families and friends (not to mention their jobs) for three months. And believe me, *these* Boot Camps are no spa; it's really, really hard work—and part of that work is coping with the emotional fallout from being away from their regular lives and thrust into a situation where they must confront their demons.

You don't have to pull a donkey up a hill to lose weight or go to any other extremes. But your chances of succeeding are exponentially higher if you have the same whatever-it-takes attitude that drives people to work out enough to burn 7,000 calories in one day. Because you can't just dabble in weight loss and expect to reach your goals. Think about it: Have you ever done anything halfway and had it go well? Doubtful. It's just as bad as going for the quick fix. So if your idea of being ready is to say, "Okay, I won't have dessert for a month, and I'll stop eating bread, but I'm not going to exercise" or "I'll go to the gym, but I refuse to give up Friday happy hour with my friends," then you're fooling yourself.

I am sure you can do an Internet search on how to lose weight without working out, or find a study on the reasons why you shouldn't restrict your calories. Whoever tells you that you don't need to do both is full of crap. You can always find some "research" or make up your own excuse to confirm whatever it is you want to do in life. But what if for once you took a different approach? Look for what scares you. Instead of looking for things you can use to talk yourself out of what you know you need to do, look inside and start being honest with how unhappy you are. Then you'll see—you'll know—that you have to be all in to get results.

And when I say "all in" I mean *all* in. It's not even okay to say, "I will follow a diet and exercise plan to the letter, but I'm not going to deal with the secret I've been holding onto for 20 years." Whether you know it or not, it's the secret that's making you eat. **What you perceive as hunger pain is really emotional pain**.

Most times, cherry-picking what you will and won't do leads to failure. Choose to ignore any of the bad habits, destructive coping techniques, rationalizations, and enabling relationships that have made you fat in the first place at your peril: You have to address all of them. The people I know who've been successful at weight loss have changed just about everything in their lives. That doesn't mean you have to do everything at once. I'm all for taking baby steps, which I'll talk about in Chapter 13. But you have to commit to doing everything it takes to get a healthier body. And consistency is everything. Showing up each day at the same time to the gym, working out hard, eating at the same time—all these factors are important. And you have to be in it for the long haul. Weeks are not enough. Months, years—essentially always—making the right decisions will not only get you to where you want to be but also will inspire others around you, including your friends, family, co-workers, and even people you've never met but who have seen you from across the gym.

I'd say that I'm a pretty disciplined exerciser, but even I'm amazed and inspired by the diligence of others. For more than a year, I would pass a guy running every day at 5:30 a.m., in the dark, on the path by my house. I would finish my 7-mile run, shower, eat breakfast, get ready for the day, drive my kid to school, and on the way back from drop-off see him just finishing his workout! Two and a half hours! I ended up seeing less and less of this guy, and by that I mean that there was less of him to see. Over that year, he had been steadily losing weight.

I was just in awe of the guy. He was keeping me motivated, but I didn't even know his name! Finally, one day I stopped him and said, "Excuse me, but I have seen you out here for the last year, and I am amazed at how hard you've been working. Do you mind if I ask you how much weight you've lost?"

He was embarrassed, and I got the feeling that he didn't want to let me know. So I told him that he had inspired me with his work ethic. He then said, "I think at last check, I have lost 160 pounds." One-hundred-and-sixty pounds! Are you kidding me? In the dark, by himself, pushing day after day, this man lost 160 pounds! His name is Sam, and now every morning, we scream and root each other on like we are long-lost brothers.

"Morning Sam! Go get 'em!"

"You saved my life, JD" (I told him I was one of the creators of *The Biggest Loser*, and it turned out that that was the show that got him to begin his journey . . . the irony!)

"You did all the work, Sam!" I say. It's a ritual I now look forward to.

I always say that, in setting any goal in life: The best backup plan is no backup plan. What kind of advice is that? Who would tell their kid, "You know what, follow your dreams of being a rock 'n' roll star or the great American novelist, and don't have a backup plan." It's sounds like horrible advice. And yet it's the advice I give everyone, every single person, especially those looking to get into the television business. It's just another way of saying that you need to be all in. In the case of aspiring showbiz folks, if you're not all in, there's going to be someone more committed than you. In the case of weight loss, leaving some wiggle room is going to just make you that much more susceptible to bagging exercise and curling up on the couch with a pint of Ben and Jerry's.

So tell yourself that you have nothing to fall back on; you have no alternative but to adopt a healthy lifestyle. You're Butch Cassidy and the Sundance Kid standing on a cliff with your nemesis fast approaching on horseback. It's jump off the cliff or perish. When you have it in your head that there's no safety net, it makes it easier to forge ahead—and that leads to success. You don't have to be perfect. This isn't about perfection. There will be cookies eaten and workouts missed; everybody screws up occasionally. But having that do-or-die mind-set will help keep you from messing up too often—as well as ensure that when you do mess up, you quickly put it behind you and return to your healthy habits. The new you is going to be defined by what you do *after* a screw-up.

2. Why are you trying to lose weight?

There's no right answer to this question. You want to look better, feel better, save your life—every one of those reasons is legitimate. You'll hear a lot of experts say things like: "Don't try and lose weight for a high-school reunion." Or a wedding. Or a tropical vacation. I don't have a problem with these slightly superficial weight-loss incentives because, while some people will just go back to their old habits once they get that reunion-presentable body, other people may find that it starts them on a life-altering path. Those things can give you a good jump-start. If putting a picture on the treadmill of the guy who broke up with you and told you were fat makes you run faster, I'm all for it. Don't worry about whether you're losing weight for the "right" reasons. Just get going, and do it.

||||||||||||||||||||||||||||||||||||||||||||||||||||||||||||||||||||||||||||

Need a Good Reason to Lose Weight? How about a Dramatic Change in Your Health?

Last year, my A1C [blood glucose level] was 7.9, bona fide diabetic. I have been a type 2 diabetic since 2003 (after the birth of my first child). Yesterday, I received my 28-page blood panel and my A1C is 6.4. That means that I am off of my medication and need to just monitor my life and levels. I'm so overjoyed; I can't stop the tears of joy. I could climb the Empire State Building on the adrenaline pumping in my nonclogged arteries.

—Nikki, posted on *The Revolution* Facebook page

I recently met a woman at the gym who'd I seen grinding it out day after day. She was quite overweight and seemed to be working like crazy to get the pounds off. "Elaine," I asked her, "why are you working so hard at it? What's your goal?" Elaine told me that she was going on a trip to Jerusalem and wanted to climb up to Masada, an ancient fortress situated on top of a high rock plateau; losing weight and getting fit were going to make it happen for her. But in our later conversations—Elaine, by the way, had no idea what I did for a living—it also came out that the climb up was really just a metaphor for climbing out of a life that had been filled with unhappiness. She had long been divorced, and her weight made her insecure in social situations. She had virtually been hiding away. In a sense, every day presented Elaine with a hill to climb, but the one in Jerusalem—that climb was going to set her free.

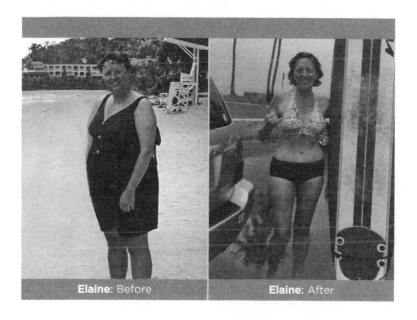

Elaine: Before   **Elaine:** After

Elaine was hoping that losing weight would help her find love—now that's a good, purposeful, meaningful reason to lose weight. But what happened to Elaine was so much bigger. Being overweight had made Elaine's life become very small. Maybe that's happened to you. The more weight you gain, the smaller and smaller your life becomes because you never venture out of your comfort zone. What shedding pounds did for Elaine was make her brave. She wanted to learn how to row, so she found a club in the marina and joined. She learned to sail. She had never been skiing before, so one day, she just hopped in her snappy convertible (she got it after she lost all the weight), drove the five hours up to the mountains, skied all the next day, and drove home. There seem to be no limits to what she'll do. That's what I'm talking about when I say that losing weight is just the beginning.

Of course, Elaine climbed up to that fortress in Jerusalem, too. But she didn't consider it the finish line. Last time I saw her was at the gym. The "new" Elaine was there an hour before her appointment with a trainer, working out harder than most anyone I know. It's worth noting that Elaine is one of the many inspiring people I have met out in the real world. Inspiring people are all around us, if we just take the time to learn their stories.

The night before the winner of the very first *The Biggest Loser* was announced, the guy in the lead—his name was Gary—went out for a normal dinner with his family and had a healthy meal, shared some laughs, talked about how happy he was about what he'd accomplished, then went to sleep. Gary's closest competitor took a different tack: He went to the gym and worked out, pushing it to the bitter end. And it paid off. He beat Gary by one pound. *One pound.* That one pound cost Gary $250,000.

You probably think I'm going to say, "Wasn't the guy who won awesome, never letting up! Isn't he the very definition of all in?" But that's not what I'm going to say. I saw Gary many years later, and he was still thin and healthy. The winner put all the weight back on. Competition is the premise behind *The Biggest Loser,* so people motivated by beating out others often win the cash. But the real winners are those whose reasons for losing weight evolve into something deeper. Gary was very upset about losing at first, but then he realized what the bigger win was. He wanted to get his life back, and he did. The other guy was in it mostly just to win it. That only got him so far.

If I had to choose a "best" reason to lose weight, it's good health. Getting back medical test results that show just how bad things have gotten has made more than a few people drastically change their eating and exercise habits. Some people, fortunately, figure it out before their doctors read them the riot act. (Just as an aside, some people have even told me that they purposefully choose doctors who are overweight, hoping that it means the doctor will not preach about adopting a healthy lifestyle since he or she obviously doesn't have one either.) One of our Season 5 *Extreme Weight Loss* cast members, Mitzi, told me that turning 52 gave her a wake-up call. "My mother passed away at age 65. When I started doing the math, I realized I wasn't too far away from it." Wanting to live a long and healthy life—what better reason for losing weight could you have?

3. Are you willing to dive into your brain and figure out why you're fat?

This is where the *The Big Fat Truth* solution to weight loss comes in. Being ready to assess your inner life is probably the hardest part of losing weight. The treadmill, the workout equipment, eating right—you can do that. Looking inside yourself, though, is like opening Pandora's box; you might not like what comes flying out. That's especially true if you've had a trauma in your past, but even if you haven't, don't kid yourself. There's something going on in your head that's preventing you from getting the best out of life.

More than likely, you're going to have to face some things you've been sweeping under the rug, and sometimes, that can be painful. Maybe you have a big secret; maybe you just have to admit to yourself that you've been self-indulgent not because of any terrible event, but because a low level of unhappiness pervades your life. What's the missing piece? Be prepared to find out and work on changing it, and you will regain jurisdiction over your body. Now might not seem like a good time to take a deep emotional dive; it never is. We're all so busy just living our lives that we forget to be introspective. And no one likes a mess—emotional stuff is messy. **But to have a breakthrough, you're probably going to have to have a few breakdowns;** it's just part of the process. So get off the hamster wheel of life for a while. Don't think about the bills, the laundry, the kids, the carpool, trying to get a promotion—those are all external things. Instead, look inward. Turn off the background noise of life and turn on the sounds of self-examination. Fall back in love with yourself, and then you are playing the game.

In the end, the things that you fear most are also the things that will help you grow. They're the things that will help you take the biggest leap forward. Without a breakdown, there is no breakthrough. As we go along, I'll talk more about this critical part of weight loss. For now, I just want to know if you're willing to find the *real* answer to the question: Why are you fat?

4. Can you imagine yourself telling other people you're trying to lose weight—and even asking them for help?

Wait—you're not going on one of my shows, so why does the world need to know what you're doing? There are a few reasons, starting with the fact that telling others what you're doing helps make you take a more honest look at yourself. When contestants on *The Biggest Loser* or *Extreme Weight Loss* weigh in, we make them take off their shirts and show the TV audience what their bodies really look like. Of course, this contributes to the drama because you can really see how radically they've changed their bodies by the end of the season; it is a TV show, after all. We're not, though, trying to humiliate or shame them. Far from it. We also ask the cast to put their fat on display because it's not just the audience that's seeing them as they really are; they are seeing themselves. You might think that by standing in line to audition for the show, our contestants have already acknowledged their problem, and, yeah, they have, sort of. But most people who don't like their bodies change and even shower in the dark; they don't really look. They don't see how bad it's gotten until it hits them smack in the face.

The very first weigh-in is the cast members' kiss-the-curb moment. By that I mean that they can't get any lower than this. It's their coming out. They're admitting in front of everyone, including themselves, that they have a problem—it's like when a drinker stands up in an AA meeting and says, "My name is John, and I'm an alcoholic." I'm not suggesting that you do the same thing in the conference room at work by coming out to unsuspecting co-workers—unless, of course, you want to! But you can make a declaration in a different way. Just make sure that you plant the flag in the ground loudly, proudly, and with conviction.

Again, you don't necessarily need to take off your shirt and put a selfie on Facebook (but if you do, I will applaud loudly!). If you're fat, people already know it. But you do need to be ready to let other people know that *you* know you have a problem, and you're working to change. Along the way, you're going to need friends and family to help you and hold you accountable, so if you're not ready to reach out, stop reading. Come back to this page when you feel you can be open and accept the help you need.

Reaching out can be scary, but let me just say this: If you're not a little afraid of what's to come, then I'd hesitate. Yes, you should be enthusiastic and raring to go, but changing your lifestyle is hard. It requires making sacrifices, including your pride. So it's okay to feel butterflies in your stomach (just don't mistake those feelings for hunger pains); in fact, you should. You're letting go of the notion that there's an easy way to lose weight and admitting to yourself that you have a lot of work ahead of you. That's tough.

One of our contestants, a young woman named Amber, who was on *Extreme Weight Loss* with her fiancé, told me that her readiness quotient went way up when she stopped thinking that there was an easy way to lose weight. "I thought I was ready when I tried CrossFit for two weeks. I thought I was ready when I went on the paleo diet and got a workout DVD. But looking back, I wasn't ready. I wanted a quick fix. I didn't want to do the work." So yes, there is going to be work to do. But don't for a minute think you can't do it, because you absolutely can.

5. Are you ready for how incredible your life is going to be?

Being overweight can take the joy out of life in both little and big ways. One thing I was surprised and sad to learn over the past few years is how many people sleep in recliners, because they've become so big it's uncomfortable to lie flat on a bed. We've had people on the show who are taking up to 20 pills a day because they have so many obesity-related problems. Even people who don't have a lot of weight to lose feel uncomfortable in their bodies—and in their too-tight clothes—plus know that they could be headed down the recliner-and-20-pills-a-day road if they don't get their eating in check. No one wants to live a life hampered by his or her body size.

I think the way Mitzi described being overweight to me sums it up well. "The weight weighs you down and makes you live a life that's small. You're big, yet your life is so small." When Mitzi attended *Extreme Weight Loss* Boot Camp, her group did a series of activities, including an obstacle course race called the Warrior Dash, six 5Ks, and whitewater rafting. "I can promise you that I never thought about going whitewater rafting. That wasn't on my radar, bucket list, nothing," she laughs.

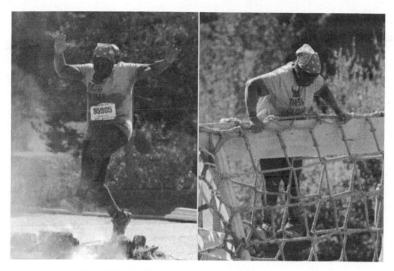

Mitzi doing a Warrior Dash and climbing ropes

And that was just the beginning. The group also went to an amusement park. "For a fat person, an amusement park is panicsville" she says. "You look for the sign that says the ride's weight capacity and hope and pray that you fall under it, and that the bar in the roller-coaster car will go down. To get to the point, after losing the weight, where I didn't have to worry about the weight capacity, and the bar just clicked into place, was joyful. I rode some rides six or seven times!"

When Mitzi thinks back to the time before she lost weight, she remembers how left out being fat could make her feel. "Some of my friends were going to do a 5K with lots of obstacles, and they never even thought to ask if I wanted to participate. They asked if I'd support them and be there as a cheerleader. The truth is, I probably couldn't have kept up or done the obstacles, but it still hurt. So I sat on the sidelines and took photos." Now, though, things are different. "I have photos of me doing a Warrior Dash. I have photos of me climbing a cargo line and jumping over a fire. It makes me feel proud. I'm not living small anymore. I'm living large in a smaller body."

* * * * *

Whether your goal is to be skinny enough to jump over fire one day, complete a marathon, slip into a slinky dress, throw your blood pressure medicine down the toilet, or just feel more comfortable in you own skin, know that it's going to happen. You'll be *living* life, not just existing—and it's going to be great.

CHAPTER 2

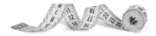

Think You Can, Think You Can't— Either Way You're Right

This is a typical conversation in my household.

"Dad, I could never get an A on that test."

"Well, you definitely just got a B or less."

"But I haven't even taken it yet!"

"You said you can't get an A, so you won't get an A. Mentally, you already took the test."

There are two types of people in the world. Those who say "I can" and those who say "I can't," and both of them are right. If you don't think you can do something, you won't be able to. "I can't" is a self-fulfilling prophecy. Think about it: Is being an "I can't" person at the heart of your failure to lose weight? That can be remedied. Be an "I can" kind of person, and you won't hope for an A, but rather demand it, expect it—and feel empowered to do the work to make it happen.

The power of the "I can" mind-set is amazing. We had a guy named Danny try out for *The Biggest Loser* who weighed more than anyone I'd ever seen at his age. He was 18 years old and weighed 450 pounds. *Four-fifty.* He couldn't even close his hands to make a fist, he was so fat. I usually think anyone can do anything, but I had my doubts about him. I was honest about it with him, too.

"You scare me," I said to him. "I don't think we can have you on the show. Honestly, I don't think you can do it. And, by the way, dude, where are your shoes?"

"It's too hard to get them on," he replied. This was the most important meeting in this kid's life, and he couldn't even get his shoes on? I felt bad for him, but told him I still didn't think he could safely master the challenges the show would put in front of him.

"Name it," he said. "I'll do anything to be on this show. How do you want me to prove that I can do it?" I couldn't tell if the desperation in his voice was genuine or if he had just rehearsed the words in his room, preparing the "Sunday Sermon" I mentioned earlier.

"Okay," I said, figuring I'd scare him off. "Go out of this room and take the first door on your right. It's the stairs. Take them down to the bottom"—we were on the 20th floor of the Sheraton Universal—"then walk back up."

Without hesitation, he walked out of the room, still shoeless, and nine other potential contestants all let out a sigh of relief that I didn't pick them. Yet there was also a sparkle in their eyes as if to say, "If he can do it, I can do it, too." Singling out one person might seem cruel, but, in fact, I've found that the one person who's picked often inspires the whole room so that, suddenly, maybe for the first time in their lives, instead of feeding on food, they start feeding off each other's positive energy.

After about 15 minutes, I started to get worried about the guy. Maybe he'd gone home. Maybe (hopefully not) he'd died halfway down. I got increasingly nervous. I went to see if I could locate him.

I finally found him on the ninth floor on his way back up, huffing and puffing, spitting and coughing all over the place. He was soaked in sweat. But he kept going, bare feet and all. When he finally made it back into the roomful of would-be contestants, he burst through the door, barely able to speak. The place erupted with applause. Standing ovation. *He did it. Barefoot.* But not only that; he made them all believe that they could do it, too. Everyone in the room had just had a moment they'd never forget. I know I did. That day, on the 20th floor of the Sheraton Universal, transformation happened right before my eyes. The kid went on to appear on the show and lost almost 250 pounds over two seasons. Now that's somebody who said to himself: "I can."

So say you only have 30 pounds to lose. Maybe only 15 pounds. How does this kid's story relate to you? First, I hope that it inspires you. That's what all the stories we tell on our shows are meant to do, and I hope the stories I tell you throughout this book do the same. If this 450-pound guy could drag himself up 20 flights of stairs barefoot, surely you can spend an hour on an elliptical trainer every day or give up grabbing a doughnut and vanilla latte each morning. But the bigger message is that you really are capable of doing things that seem impossible to you.

I know that you hold some habits very dear. And that things can *seem* complicated. You've been accompanying colleagues to the Mexican place around the corner from your office for eight years. You can't just stop going; they'd think you don't like them anymore. You're so busy that it's all you can do to get macaroni and cheese from a box, pizza from your regular delivery place, or take-out Chinese on the table for your family each night. How are you going to feed everyone if you give up that fat-promoting, artery-clogging menu? But look around you. Real friendships withstand changes in eating habits, and there are many quick-fix dinners that don't involve a load of grease and calories (or money). All it takes is a belief that you can change. If you think you can, then you will find the solutions to your problems.

When people protest that they aren't capable of doing something, I see it as a challenge to convince them that they can. And I relish it. I want to get inside their heads and help them get rid of their kryptonite.

"Tell me what you can't live without," I'll ask cast members.

"I could never live without my chocolate cake."

"Great. You just committed to me that, for one year, you're not going to eat any chocolate cake. You over there. You say you can't live without diet soda? Great, you are never going to drink diet soda again."

I make it my mission to show cast members that the things they think they can't live without actually have no power over them. I'll put a cake on the table, open up the box, and let the smell of chocolate fill the air. As they sit down to eat all their meals, they'll smell that chocolate wafting by. It's called exposure therapy, and it sounds like torture, but ask anyone who's been through it—it just speeds up the process. You sit down for every meal next to a chocolate cake and don't stick your finger in to have even one lick of frosting, and soon you'll be able to give up lots of things you never thought you could.

Sometimes, you just need proof that you really *can* do something you believe you can't. I got so tired of hearing people on *The Biggest Loser* say, "I can't run, I'm not a runner," that I decreed, "okay, every finalist on this show is going to run a full marathon." You should have seen the panic on their faces. Every medical professional, every standards-and-practice person at the network said, "You can't do that."

"We can and we will," I told them. All four of our finalists not only ran the full 26.2 miles, they set the bar for contestants to come. Think about it. These people went from not being able to run one mile to running 26.2 miles in less than six months. Again it proves that **the body is no match for the power of the mind.** Say that last sentence out loud. Again. Say it until you believe it! *You* tell your body what to do, and if it doesn't listen, tell it again until it does. Your mind will get you over this perceived mountain, but not without the conviction it takes to fight the battle every minute of every day. Where are you fat? *In your head!* Your body is just the outcome!

|||||||||||||||||||||||||||||||||||||||||||||||||||||||||||||||||||||||||||||||||||||||

What Would It Feel Like to Be Living in a Different Body, with a Different Mind-Set?

JD,

I watched your TEDx talk [http://tedxtalks.ted.com/video/You-Don-t-See-What-I-See-%7C-JD-R] today and found myself sobbing uncontrollably at my desk. I began sobbing harder when I saw how much space I had between the armrests of my desk chair and my thighs. The last time I sat in this chair was before Boot Camp, and I had to adjust the arm rests to keep them from cutting into my legs. My goodness, how things have changed.

I felt an incredible sense of accomplishment when I heard you mention that you could tie a doughnut around many of the people on the show's neck and they wouldn't eat it. I realized . . . I'm that person! I wouldn't eat a doughnut right now if you attached it to me, and paid me to eat it. Then I thought, Why wouldn't I eat it? Is it because I have a weigh-in next Monday and a deadline to meet, or because I've transformed enough to know what's best for me and what isn't? Would I refuse the doughnut because I'm afraid of a camera over my shoulder or because nothing (not even that doughnut) would taste as good as all the extra room in my desk chair feels? I felt so proud because I realized I wouldn't eat the doughnut for the right reasons!!

—Hannah, *Extreme Weight Loss* cast member, via email

The "I can't" mind-set isn't unique to people who are overweight. Skinny people have just as hard a time giving things up. They're not special. They basically have the same brain as you do and the same issues to deal with. Taking the naturally thin people out of the equation, most people who are skinny just exercise greater willpower. They say, "I can" eat healthfully, "I can" exercise hard, and they do.

Let's be clear about the difference between "can't" and "don't want to." If you think you can't do something, it means that there is a brief moment when you contemplated it. "Can I? Nah, I can't." Maybe if you'd paused just a little longer you would have seen that what you were really saying was not "I can't," but "I don't want to." Ask yourself what it is you believe. Can you not do something or do you just not want to? Not wanting to is a choice; thinking you're not capable is a mind-set—a mind-set that you can change if you see yourself accomplish what you once thought was impossible.

There are going to be plenty of times—especially when it comes to exercise—where your body tells you, *Hey, I can't do that.* But if your mind says you can, eventually, your body will listen. Just when you think you can't do another push-up, that voice in your head—*Do I want to be the person who can or the person who can't?*—will help you fight on. And don't just do one more. Do 10 more. Go *past* the goal to prove to yourself that it's just a number. On a treadmill, 5.5 miles per hour is just a number. If 5.5 mph is your goal, go to 6.0 mph to confirm that a number does not define you.

This isn't just the old mind-over-matter argument. There are actually some sport scientists investigating the possibility that the muscle fatigue we feel when exercising hard does not really signal that your muscles are going to fail—in fact, you're probably only using about 40 percent of your muscles' capacity when working out hard. The fatigue you feel may just be the body's way of conserving energy. It doesn't mean that you are incapable of doing more. So when you feel that you can't take another step, know that you actually can: You have the physical potential; it's just not being unlocked by your mind.

Panda (the nickname everyone knows him by) is a young guy who definitely believed he was incapable of losing weight. Yet, as it turns out, he so excelled at paring down that he reached his goal in three months. On *Extreme Weight Loss*, we give people a year to lose weight; Panda lost all the weight he needed to while still in

Boot Camp. It was monumental. One hundred pounds, obliterated. I bring up Panda because, initially, he had a striking lack of the "I can" factor. Tellingly, he was nicknamed after a lazy animal that sleeps most of the day. We get people on our shows that are as confident in their abilities as can be—"I can do this, just show me how"—but Panda considered himself a 90-pound weakling (who just happened to be carrying another 230 pounds).

Panda had tried out for *The Biggest Loser* and made it to the semifinals one year, but ultimately got sent home. Still, we remembered him, and when it came time to cast Season 5 of *Extreme Weight Loss,* we called him back in. Korean by birth, but raised in an adoptive American family, he had been physically abused by his older brother and was carrying the burden of having never told his loving-but-clueless adoptive parents the extent of the mistreatment he'd suffered. Panda works as a camp counselor, a job he adores but describes as like being a parent to 12 kids 24 hours a day, 7 days a week. In other words, it's stressful, giving him the perfect excuse to soothe himself with food. Add to that the fact that he has a nickname that equates him with a big, round, cuddly animal, and Panda just got larger and larger.

There was another problem, too. Panda was inclined to think of himself as incapable of change. "I always felt like I was too weak to lose weight," says Panda. "I wasn't strong enough mentally to do it. Part of that comes from living in a pretty broken home and learning to be submissive and give up my needs. That reinforced that I didn't have any willpower."

That feeling of weakness pervaded Panda's life. He wasn't strong enough to tell his parents about his brother's abuse, and he wasn't strong enough to resist enticing foods that he knew were bad for him. His weakness was reinforced when he tried a number of diets and found he couldn't stay on them. "I started doing radical things. I went on the Atkins Diet. I became a vegetarian, then a vegan with a side of bacon, which turned into the I'll-only-eat-meat-on-weekends diet," he recalls. "Then I started doing diet pills, which had horrible side effects. It all just contributed to the idea that I was weak."

This is the same guy that lost about a third of his body weight in three months so, in fact, he's not weak—he just needed the opportunity to prove it to himself. But what's especially heartening about Panda's story is that he eventually gathered up the strength to talk to his parents about things he had bottled up inside for years. This is exactly what I'm talking about when I say that dropping pounds can change your life in amazing ways. "The weight-loss process proved to me that I was strong, and not just physically strong," says Panda, "but mentally strong. Mental strength is a lot harder to build. I think our minds might just be the weakest muscle we have." To me, that was such a deep thought. It was the first time I have ever heard someone say that, and it makes complete sense. Work out that muscle and your problems will be solved!

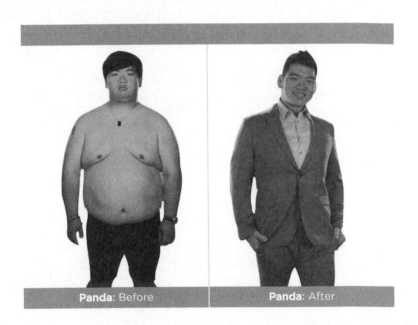

Panda: Before   Panda: After

When you say "I can" to resisting a cookie, and "I can" to running a 5K race, and "I can" to telling your friends that you don't want to eat at Greasy Joe's Rib Shack anymore, it's just a small leap to being able to say "I can" quit this lousy job and "I can" tell my spouse that I want to be treated better and "I can" follow my dream of becoming an artist. It just bleeds into every part of your life. When you become an "I can" person, every glass becomes half full and life improves exponentially.

Let me just tell you one more story about someone who has an unbelievable can-do spirit. We had a contestant on *The Biggest Loser*, Moses, who blew out his knee within the first week of the show. He couldn't do anything that required being on his feet, which meant no running, no walking—there really was very little that he could do to burn calories. And that was a big problem because, in order to stay on that show, you have to drop pounds each week. *The Biggest Loser* is all about the weigh-in. Moses also did not want to let down his daughter Kaylee, his partner on the show. But in my opinion, he was done; we were about to eliminate him.

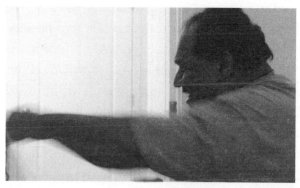

Moses shadowboxing

So what does this guy do? Fold? A few weeks before he might have played the victim card and said that it was through no fault of his own that he couldn't continue. But not this time. This time, he came up with the idea of sitting on the edge of his bed and shadow boxing for *12* hours a day. Some switch in this guy's mind had flipped, making unbelievable commitment possible. Sweat poured off him in rivers. The bed was soaking wet. He definitely didn't say, "I can't." That's what most people would say. Here's what I say: If you want something, you will figure out how to get it, just like the shadow boxer did. Desire leads to bright ideas. Put another way, desperation is the greatest motivator.

It helps, too, if you start thinking of yourself as someone who is powerful, competent, and capable of extraordinary things. You are!

To me, one of the most inspiring guys ever was the college basketball coach Jimmy Valvano, who sadly died of cancer at the age of 43. In one motivational speech he gave, Valvano tells the story of how, as a 16-year-old at basketball camp, he heard a pastor he admired say, "The Lord must have loved ordinary people because he made so many of us." That disheartened Valvano—he had thought he was special! But then the pastor went on to say that, "every single day, in every walk of life, ordinary people accomplish extraordinary things." That became Valvano's rallying cry: You don't have to be some spectacularly talented person with a will of steel to do something remarkable. *It's not extraordinary people who do extraordinary things; it's ordinary people who do extraordinary things.* That can be you. That *is* you. Just add the word "extra" to your "ordinary" life, and go do something amazing.

The people I talk about in this book who changed their lives are no different from you. They are ordinary people with ordinary families and ordinary jobs. What sets them apart is that they believed that they could do something extraordinary. This can-do confidence doesn't happen overnight. Nobody goes from lying on the couch eating a whole coffee cake to the perfect life in 24 hours. Most people get there by taking baby steps. Each small victory you accomplish gets you one step closer to becoming an "I can" person.

If you say, "I can keep my promises," you'll take a step forward. "I can choose to have a better life for myself." Take a step forward. "I can make decisions that will give me that better life." Take another step forward. Pretty soon all of those baby steps add up to something amazing. Suddenly, instead of giving up before you even get started, you'll start seeing obstacles as inspiration. Like that guy who shadow boxed for 12 hours a day, you'll be unstoppable. By the way, have you ever tried to shadow box in your bed for even 12 minutes? I have. It's exhausting—and he did it for 12 hours! The power of the mind still amazes me each day.

CHAPTER 3

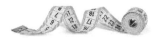

Listen to What (the Right) People Are Trying to Tell You

I don't have to tell you that fat people, especially fat kids, are prime targets for cruelty. No doubt someone—maybe even lots of people—have said something mean to you about your weight. And it's awful. The pain and self-hatred these insults dredge up are hard to bear. It's enough to make you build the Great Wall of Chinese food around your heart so that nothing anybody says about your body, your eating habits, and your general neglect of your health can penetrate. But that's a problem. If you tune out everyone, when people who love and care about you try to tell you the hard truth about yourself, you're going to shut them down, too.

Instead, you're going to listen to those people who want you to stay fat and unhealthy either because they like you the way you are or (the more likely reason) because they need a partner in doughnut and pizza crimes. "Yeah, they're right," they have you saying to yourself, "there's nothing wrong with me."

These are not people who truly want the best for you. They're nonfriend friends. Not only do they not help you come to the critical realization that you need to change but also they make you feel that staying the way you are is the best way to win people's love and affection. This is something just about every cast member on our show has grappled with. "I thought that my body and the way I ate was what people appreciated about me," says Bruce, who is one of our best *Extreme Weight Loss* success stories. "It's not okay for people to take drugs. People hide them, and society frowns on them. With eating, it's okay. You can go out and have dinner and feel good about yourself. So I could eat as much food as I wanted to eat. Everyone searches for acceptance, and I think I thought that was the way I was accepted. It's cliché but true—I was the good-time guy. 'Oh, Bruce is here, he'll eat all the food.' I thought that was okay." For Bruce, his ability to chow down was like a badge of honor.

"Bru-u-u-u-uce! Bruce will eat it."

"Hell, yes, I'll eat it. I'm the man!"

Panda, the young cast member I mentioned earlier, said he often told himself that he was happy being the size he was. "People like me at this size. I don't intimidate people. This is how people know me, and this is how I have to be for them," he'd say to himself. What he admits now: "That was a fake mask I was wearing."

While the people who want you to stay just the way you are may love you, they love themselves more. Or at least they don't want their way of life threatened. If you change, what's that going to say about them? It might say that they, too, need to change, something they're simply not up for. Also, they often don't want what they see as your personality—who they *think* you are—to change. Believe it or not, even friends and families of alcoholics can fear what will happen when they're loved one gets sober. It's fear of the unknown. Will that person who gets healthy become a proselytizer? Or maybe end up just plain dull? Suddenly, the life of the party is gone; nobody wants that.

Besides the fact that someone's health is more important than the amusement of others, that's just idiotic. I've seen lots of life-of-the-party types drop half their weight and still be just as engaging as ever. And without their bodies weighing on their minds, I've even seen some people who frankly weren't that interesting before come out of their shells to become some of the most fun people ever. Regardless of the outcome, you cannot let other people's fears and desires drag you down. It's time we retired the old fat-people-are-jolly line. Most of the fat people I know are in pain. When they're alone, they're far from jolly.

Still, I get why people equate eating behavior and/or body shape with identity. Would Melissa McCarthy and John Goodman have such outsized personalities if their bodies weren't outsized? Would Barbara Streisand still sell records without that nose? If I couldn't eat healthfully and exercise, I wouldn't feel like myself, so it goes both ways. We'd all probably still be the same people at our core if we went through physical changes, but it's hard to visualize it if you're used to seeing someone—or yourself—a certain way.

A few years ago, a famous comedian was all set to join one of our weight-loss shows. He came to me and said he was finally ready to lose the weight because he was the only person he knew over 400 pounds and 60 years old. I told him that it was because all the others are dead. I was very excited for him and got the network to agree to have him on the show. I called him to say congratulations and could hear his nervous laugh over the phone. He said, "I guess this means I really have to do it now, huh?" I knew right then and there it was going to end badly.

He went through all of the medical testing anyway and moved into the cast accommodations, ready to start Boot Camp. But as I'd expected, it didn't start well. On the very first day of Boot Camp, he actually asked if he was going to have to do the same thing as the other people. "Yes!" I screamed. The following day, he asked to be driven to the gym—which was less then a half-mile away—even as he watched the other 13 participants start their walk over. He was not ready to do the work needed to push past the pain and fear and improve on his life. He was too worried about what he would lose (and I am not talking about pounds). In the end, he just couldn't do it. He moved out after a week. His biggest fear was that losing weight would make people think he wasn't funny anymore. He had spent the better part of his life trading on his size. If he lost that, how would he make money? "People aren't going to laugh at my jokes the same way. I'm the funny fat guy," he said.

Yeah, but was that really his fear? Or was it that *he* didn't think he would be funny if he reduced his more-than-400 pound size? Actually, he might have been even funnier if he mined that dark side of himself for humor rather than making fun of his size. But we'll never know: He was an "I can't" kind of guy. I tried to tell him that it would be a rebirth of his career. "Think of the press you will get!" Still, I couldn't get through to him.

Raymond and Robert, twins who appeared on Season 5, were a lot like Bruce, the *Extreme Weight Loss* cast member I introduced you to earlier. They also had part of their identity rooted in their friends' ideas of them. "Don't lose weight, man," their friends would say any time one of them would try a little self-improvement— even though they both weighed nearly 400 pounds. "Your size is part of your personality. You are big, funny guys."

But they also had friends who told them differently, especially their best friend, Chris. But it took a while for his words to get through. He'd say to them, "You guys have to do something, you guys are fat."

"What?" they'd say back to him, offended.

"Yeah, you guys are fat. As long as I've known you, you've never been this big. You have let yourselves go, and you have to change."

During the initial casting of *Extreme Weight Loss*, potential cast members start the weight-loss process, and then go home for a while (if they're picked for the show) before starting Boot Camp. When the twins returned home from casting, they went to see Chris, thinking he'd be impressed (they'd lost about 20 pounds

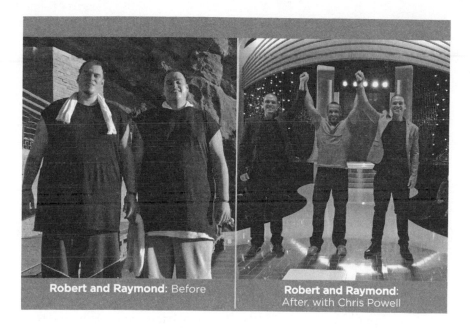

Robert and Raymond: Before

Robert and Raymond: After, with Chris Powell

each in only two weeks—a great start). Instead he said, "I kind of thought you'd be smaller." Ouch! And I know, it seems kind of mean and unsupportive, but, fortunately, the twins didn't take it that way. "He tells us straight up and calls us out on everything," says Robert. "At first it kind of pisses you off, but at least you know he's not going to sugarcoat it." This is why Robert and Raymond were ultimately successful. They were open to listening and didn't let negative comments get in the way of their mission.

Remember Amber, from Chapter 1? The woman who came on the show with her fiancé? She, too, had people in her life telling her like it is—she just didn't want to hear it. Amber, who was 273 pounds at her highest weight, says, "I look back, and I think about those moments when both friends and family tried to sneak into my life and help me but I strong-armed them away. Someone would say, 'Amber, I think you might have a problem with food, you might be a food addict' and I would just blast them. I'm not someone who gets in people's faces, but I was so sensitive." (Amber, by the way, lost 94 pounds.)

||||||||||||||||||||||||||||||||||||||||||||||||||||||||||||||||||||||||||||

Nothing Tastes as Good as
the Right Words at the Right Time

I took my daughter to get a haircut, and she asked for Taco Bell (usually our dirty little secret when it is just us). I got her a taco and a Meximelt. Nothing for me—I didn't even try to smell it! Got home and made a salad with grilled chicken and veggies. My daughter walked though the kitchen and said, "Go Mom, I'm proud of you!" in her teenager way. I cannot express how good that made me feel!

—Amy, posted on *The Revolution* Facebook page

Everyone needs someone like Amber's friends or a Chris—that is, an honest and supportive person—in his or her life; someone to hold you accountable. If you just want "yes" people to tell you how great you are, you'll never rise above your issues. I'll talk more about friends and family later, but right now, I just want to encourage you to start reconsidering the people who may have seemed a little mean and judgmental in the past. Try to see them in a different way. Maybe they were the ones who were actually trying to help you—and, most important, will be there to support you when you start making changes in your life. Of course, some of them *are* just mean and judgmental, and you don't need them. But some of them are undoubtedly worried about your well-being. Find those people that care—and who won't let you make excuses for yourself—and keep them close.

Keep in mind that the people who support you may do so in different ways, and you may need to figure out which type of friend works best for you. If you're thin-skinned, but motivated by praise, find the friend who's going to be gentle about telling you what they think is going wrong, then act as a cheerleader throughout the weight-loss process. If you need a challenge to light a fire under you, find the friend who's going to get on your case if you blow it. But also, stay open. You may be surprised to find that the type of help you think you need is actually the opposite of what will work. So try everything until you see yourself starting to respond. Most of all, turn a deaf ear to those friends who don't want you to change, and start listening to those who care for your well-being. They're going to be your lifeline throughout this process.

I suggest you also start opening up to people who are dropping subtle hints that they have information to share with you or might even be willing to lend some support. As you would expect, as soon as people find out what I do for a living, they often solicit my advice. And as you would also expect, I love to give it! But I never just thrust advice on anyone before gauging how open he or she is to hearing what I might have to say.

Not long ago, I was invited to an ABC promotional event held in honor of mommy bloggers. The network had brought 25 authors of parenting blogs to Hollywood to give them the full Disney experience, which included meeting some of ABC's television stars and executives (Disney owns ABC). I sat down at my table of bloggers to promote *Extreme Weight Loss*, but instead, it turned into something much more meaningful. I started out talking about the latest group of contestants, hoping they'd write about how successful we are at helping people lose weight, but quickly the conversation turned to *their* weight loss.

Most of the mommy bloggers were overweight themselves, and many had made the wrong decision at the buffet. Plates of tortilla chips, burritos with extra cheese, and Cokes and Diet Cokes littered our table. They began plying me for information: What should I eat? Tell me five things I can do to lose weight. One of the mommy bloggers at the table was, in fact, a daddy blogger. The lone guy among the women, he was about 100 pounds overweight. The minute he showed that he was open to discussion, I began to talk to him in earnest. "I'm betting you're not happy with your weight and that you wish you could do something about it, but it seems overwhelming," I said to him as he nodded knowingly. "I'm betting, too, that you're watching your kids pick up on the same habits you have." It wasn't long before the daddy blogger was in tears. "Okay, here's what I want you to do. . . ."

Maybe you won't find yourself sitting next to a producer of a weight-loss reality show at lunch, but you may sit next to people who've shed pounds themselves, or who help other people lose weight through exercise or diet. If they seem interested in you, take advantage of it. You'll be amazed at how much people like to help. After I gave the daddy blogger some tips, hugged him, and took his business card, I followed up with him a week later. "How's it going? Don't forget, you're adding a walk in during week two. I know it's going to be hard, but you can do it." I really wanted him to be successful, and I kept in touch. But this is not a quality unique to me. There are lots of people in the world willing to speak the truth, lend an ear, and offer you their ideas.

Mitzi, from *Extreme Weight Loss* Season 5, told me that she regretted not being more open about her problems. When she decided to come on the show, Mitzi had to tell her boss why she had to take a hiatus from her work at a nonprofit organization that helps homeless families. The woman said she was glad that Mitzi told her the reason, but also sad that she hadn't come forth earlier and asked for help. "Here I was working for an organization that helps people, but I couldn't come forth to ask for my own help," says Mitzi. "That was an eye-opener. You realize that you are hurting others because they want to help you, they want to support you." I agree. Let your defenses down, and you'll open yourself up to all the possibilities out there.

CHAPTER 4

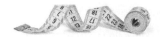

Failure and Drama Can No Longer Be Your Happy Place

How about I punch you in the face? Boom! Most people would say . . . no! Many of the people I work with love it. At least they love getting slammed in the face with words and other forms of mistreatment. It's their happy place. "I knew I couldn't get that job," "I don't deserve a raise," "that guy is too good for me," and the list goes on and on. Getting treated badly has become normal, so normal that they've not only come to expect it, they like it. It's familiar, as comforting as the frozen breakfast burrito belly bomb they eat every morning. And even though the blows are as awful as the taste of that breakfast burrito, they've come to love it in a strange kind of way, believing that it's all they deserve. What about you? Have you gotten used to the metaphorical punch in the face? Then your head is in the wrong place. We need to crack that code . . . *now!*

A few years ago, I created and executive produced a show called *I Used to Be Fat* for MTV. The premise was that by helping kids lose weight over the summer before they started college, we could help them enter their new schools as the kids they'd always wanted to be. After all, the people they were about to meet had never known them as "the fat kid." These kids had been made fun of their whole lives; we wanted to give them a fresh start.

At the end of the first day of the show, after their very first workout, I asked the 18 cast members if they were psyched. "Is there anyone that doesn't want to be here? Hold up your hand. Because I don't want to spend time and energy on you for the next 100 days if you aren't excited about it."

A boy named José instantly put up his hand. "Yeah," he said. "This isn't for me. This has been the hardest day of my life. I want no part of this. I'm out."

Moments like this are what I live for. Believe me, the other 17 kids were thinking of raising their hands, too, but couldn't muster up the courage. Or the strength—their arms were already sore from the first day's workout. I got ready to deliver some tough love to José, which would also let me remind the other 17 what a great opportunity was sitting right in front of them.

I could tell right off the bat that José was a kid who was used to failing. He didn't even want to *try* to succeed; he was just so comfortable with the status quo. But we'd given him one of our best trainers, and I wasn't about to give up. "But you have Joey, the most bad-ass trainer around! It's going to happen for you. You're going to do great," I told him.

"Nope, I'm out," he said.

This gave the other kids a perfect chance to rally around him, but the room was silent. Cue the *Rocky* music; I was about to go all out. Here's what I told him:

You get one chance to change your life. This is that chance. If it passes now, you may never get it again. Your life will always be *before* this show started and *after* it ended. Make it an "after" you can be proud of. If you can do this, anything is possible. If you can do this, you can be anything! One hundred days seems like forever, but at Day 100 when you feel like Superman, it will be worth it. Don't leave today; if you still feel this way tomorrow, then you can leave.

Within 24 hours, José was on board to stay. I never had to ask him if he wanted to leave again. He decided that day that he was going to commit and give it his all.

|||||||||||||||||||||||||||||||||||||||||||||||||||||||||||||||||||||||||||||||||||

Happy Can Be Your Happy Place

Hi JD,

I just wanted to send you a picture of my latest milestone in life! Trying on my first bikini. Life has been so amazing! It was so exhilarating to do something I never thought in a million years I could do.

—Amanda, *The Biggest Loser* contestant, via email

What he didn't anticipate was that "his all" was not only good enough but it was beyond that of any other kid participating in the show. José ended up losing 117 pounds in less then 100 days and was the most successful kid on the whole show. By taking a risk and venturing out of his happy place, he had given himself a different life. Just to give you an idea of how badly he had been treated in high school, his nickname was "Titties." No joke. Every time someone called him that, he felt defeated. It's much easier to eat that third doughnut after someone calls you a name like that. Why not eat it? You're already disgraced by your nickname. Once the show was over, though, it was a different story. His friends changed his nickname to "Pecs." Happy became his happy place.

My favorite part of the story was the final interview we had with him. He told us that for the first time in his life, he had dreams. Dreams of being successful. Dreams of being a good son. Dreams of getting a good job and making a life for himself. Just by taking control and turning a negative into a positive, his whole outlook on life changed—in 100 days! Aren't you worth that?

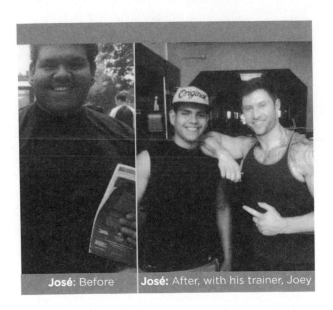

José: Before   **José:** After, with his trainer, Joey

I tell you this story because I wish I could come to your house and yell at you, too! Don't continue to let unhappy be your happy place. If I were to sit down with you and ask if you loved failure or trauma or being verbally abused by your family or boss, I'm sure you'd say no. But if any of these things are recurring in your life, you have to take a closer look and ask yourself if maybe you've become just a little too in love with misery. Maybe it's even become part of your identity.

Jennifer is a woman we had on *Extreme Weight Loss* who defined herself by her sad story. And make no mistake; she really did have a sad story. When Jennifer was 9 years old, she was playing with her younger half-brother when he fell and hit his head on the hearth in the family living room. He died three days later. It was about that time that Jennifer's stepfather, blaming her for the death, began to beat her regularly, finally driving her out of the house at age 16. (She later learned that her brother had died of spinal meningitis—the head injury had nothing to do with his death, a fact her parents knew but never told her.) The drama in Jennifer's life continued. She nearly died after a rafting incident, survived cancer three times, then married a man—her second husband and the love of her life—who she knew before the wedding was terminally ill with an autoimmune disease. Because his time was short, he had asked her to try out for the show so she could lose weight, get healthy, and be around to walk their daughters down the aisle one day. It wasn't surprising to me that Jennifer also spends her days immersed in trauma: She's a 911 operator. After reading this paragraph, you would have to agree that Jennifer had been set up to fail by her family—and by herself!

After I heard Jennifer's story, I asked her if she knew her hus-

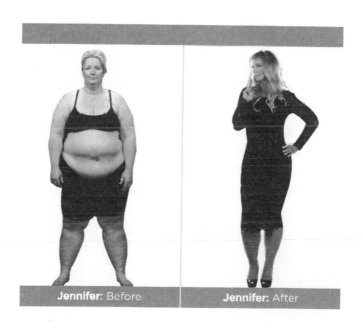

Jennifer: Before   Jennifer: After

band was sick when she married him. She said yes, and as she did, I could see her bristle. "I don't mean that you don't love him, I'm sure you do," I said to her, and she relaxed a little, "but I just wondered why you put yourself in a position that would inevitably be traumatic. You chose and had children with a man whose life, you know, is going to be cut very short. And why do you work at a job that puts you in the middle of trauma every day?"

Jennifer admitted that my questions pissed her off. I even asked her why she didn't confront her stepfather. He didn't, after all, have power over her anymore. She was making a choice to give him power over her. "The idea that it was on me, not my stepfather, made me squirm," recalls Jennifer, "but I came to realize that I didn't want to be in that victim state anymore. My sad stories had come to define me; they were who I was. I had to step out of my comfort zone and be different, and that was hard."

This is an extreme case, but an important one to look at. On a scale of 1 to 10, where do you fall on the unhappy-is-my-happy-place continuum? If you're on it at all, start thinking about why. Try to self-diagnose. What is it about the drama that sucks you in like a magnet? If you've become comfortable living in failure world, then you're inevitably going to fail at weight loss. Whether your conscious of it or not, that cozy little spot where nothing is ventured and nothing (except more pounds) is gained has come to suit you. Remember, this is a game of chess you are playing, and you have to be five moves ahead if you are going to be successful.

Start believing that failure is no longer an option for you. Resist it, repel it, use Wonder Woman wristbands to deflect it if you have to, but from this moment on, when you feel drama coming on . . . run! (Which will burn calories, too!)

CHAPTER 5

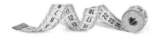

Stop Looking out the Window and Look in the Mirror

I tell every single contestant on all of our weight-loss shows the same thing. In life, to be successful, you have to have the window and the mirror. I am sure you are thinking this is some kind of L.A. new-age psychobabble, but read on. The window is the dream. It's what's out there if you could just get your act together. It's all the possibilities. What am I going to look like when I'm thin? What will life be like? Nothing wrong with picturing the future, but while, sure, the view out the window is nice, it's also not real . . . yet. The window is a passive experience. Life is *lived* in the mirror. The mirror represents action. It can sometimes cause lots of pain, but looking in the mirror can also provide the greatest moments of growth.

Everyone has to have hopes and dreams. *Realizing* your hopes and dreams is another story. You can't just spend your days dreaming about how you want your life to be, or your dreams will be just that: dreams, not reality. Too many people, I find, focus so hard on their aspirations (the window) that they ignore who they are (the mirror) and the way they're living right now. So stop looking out the window all day and start looking in the mirror. If you haven't gotten serious about losing weight until now, it's a sign that you've been looking out the window for too long.

I know why you've been avoiding the mirror. When you look in the mirror, it's easy to see how out of control you've let your life get. It's what you really look like. It's how unhealthy you probably are. And it's what you're doing to make yourself that way. Who wants to look at that? Especially with the lights on! But you have to learn to invite those moments in. As unbearable as looking at that reflection in the mirror may feel, you need to be looking at it constantly. It may be difficult to believe now, but once you start to make changes in your lifestyle, looking in the mirror will become more exciting than looking out the window. It will even improve the view out the window by helping you dream even bigger—but this time, with a real chance of making those dreams come true.

Don't just glance in the mirror—look! Act as if you're attached to a lie detector and make a truthful assessment. Pretend you are in a room with mirrors all around you; there's no way you cannot really see yourself as you are. The falsehoods will bounce off the glass and come back and hit you in the face. Truth is essential. You're never going to live that life you see out the window unless you take a good, hard look in the mirror. That's where the real work is done.

|||||||||||||||||||||||||||||||||||||||||||||||||||||||||||||||||||

A Beautiful Reflection

JD,

I found my window and my mirror, and let me tell ya, the future's lookin' bright ;).

—Tiffany, *Extreme Weight Loss* cast member, via email

What are you looking at? Not just your body. How about the way you live? Truthfully, how much are you eating? How little are you moving? What triggers your biggest binges? What issues in your life are you not dealing with? Write it all down. I want a report. And, yes, literally look in the mirror and assess your body, too, turning up the lights as bright as they will go. That might seem like a waste of time—*I know I'm fat, JD, I'm reading your book*— but you'd be surprised at how many times people come on our shows and, even though they obviously want to lose weight, they don't even realize how much they've let themselves go. Remember how I said that we make all our cast members strip down to skimpy workout wear so that they (and everyone else) can see the reality of the situation—and that some of them kind of thought things weren't so bad? It's the moment of truth; there's no hiding the bulges and rolls.

So here's what I want you to do. Look at yourself naked in the mirror and get a snapshot in your mind. Better yet, take an actual "before" photograph of you without your shirt on if you're a man and in a sports bra if you're a woman. Make an honest assessment of what you're really dealing with. Then use that picture to inspire you—not to beat yourself up. That's not the point of all this. Yes, you want to face up to what you've been doing wrong. But it's more important to use what you see to help you get excited about what you're now going to do right! The truth is, you probably know deep down that you've been eating to bury your feelings, and sweeping all the issues you need to deal with under the rug. You're unhappy. But just for now. You're going to find happiness—I know it.

Unfortunately, it's not as easy to hold a mirror up to your inner life as it is to your exterior. I've found, though, that one reliable clue to inner turmoil is the state of a person's bedroom. Sounds totally unrelated, I know, but hear me out. You could be perfectly disciplined in most areas of your life. You're, for instance, never late for work and never miss a deadline. You dress nicely, always bring the perfect gift when invited to a friend's house for dinner, and never miss the follow-up thank-you call. But in other areas of your life, you lack discipline—and you can see it plain as day in your bedroom, that most private of rooms. I have gone into cast members' bedrooms and seen more crap piled up than you can imagine. Boxes to the ceiling, a years' worth of unopened mail, dirty clothes, shoes, books, papers, dishes, cups, and fast-food wrappers scattered so thick, there's barely room to move. Sure, it's not the same for everyone. Some people, skinny or fat, are just sloppy at home. No big deal. But clutter in a private space can also be a symptom of a mind too cluttered to contend with doing stuff like eating healthfully and exercising like you're supposed to. Your bedroom should be a meditative place of calm and organization. When it's not, the first thing you see when you open your eyes in the morning is a life out of control. As soon as you start your day, your subconscious has taken over, and you're defeated.

So what's your bedroom looking like these days? Take a peek, and you'll get a good idea of who you are at this very moment. Go ahead: put this book down and spend ten minutes in silence just looking around. What is your bedroom telling you? That it's time to change?

The process of holding up a mirror to yourself also involves calling yourself out on lies. Not only lies that you tell other people but also, and most important, lies that you tell yourself. "I only ate a little bit of the ice cream." "There aren't that many calories in a cheesy Caesar salad—it's lettuce!" "I worked out for a full hour." "My ankle feels a little shaky so I better not go for a walk." *I'm* not going to lie: A large percentage of our cast members constantly deceive themselves. We hear things like, "I'm not losing weight because I don't think I'm eating enough calories." Technically, it's possible—if you cut way, way back on calories, your metabolism, in order to protect your body, can slow to a near standstill. But how often is that the case? Practically never. We also hear a lot of "I'm eating too much healthy food." Do you know what it would take to eat 2,500 calories in lettuce and carrots?

Occasionally, they tell blatant lies not only to themselves but also to us.

During a recent show, we did surveillance on a father, Jeff, and his daughter, Juliana, to see how they were doing when no one was around (remember, this is reality TV—we want to see what's real). What Chris and Heidi, a married couple and the trainers that host *Extreme Weight Loss,* witnessed was so at odds with what the father and daughter were telling them that it was shocking. For instance, Juliana, a teenager, told us on camera that she walked home from school when, in fact, she covered the distance by taking two buses, then getting a ride in a car. It took her more energy to cheat than it would have to have actually walked home! We also got photos of her carrying one of those crazy-high-calorie drinks out of Starbucks—yet she told us that she'd been perfect when it came to following her calorie limitations. Jeff said he was going to the gym when he was really going to a bakery. And these are just a few of the lies they told. They were so good at lying that they convinced themselves they were sticking with the program.

The worst part of it all was that Juliana had to witness her dad lie to the very people who were trying to help him. The behavior he modeled for his daughter made it okay for her to do the very same thing. These are not bad people, but they were doing something bad to themselves and didn't want to face up to it. When we confronted them with the evidence, they were mortified, but, to their credit, they said they weren't quitting. They had already lost quite a bit of weight, so they'd proven they were capable of doing the work; they just had to get back to it. Later on, Jeff sent me an email telling me that getting caught in a lie was his "aha moment." Better yet, knowing that he couldn't trust himself completely, he made a plan to hold himself accountable. Here's what he wrote to me:

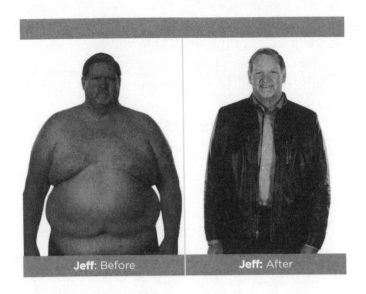

Jeff: Before   **Jeff**: After

To make sure this never happens again, any time in the future that I don't work out for at least three hours or don't eat the proper nutrition, I will confess it to my wife and daughter first, and then to you, Chris and Heidi, as well. I am going to record each day what I do and what I eat so that if at any time any of you want to know what I have been doing, I will have it readily available to show you. This will also allow me to track my weight loss better, and if I have a good or bad week, I can see what I did to cause the results.

Jeff got back to business and ended up losing a lot of weight (so did his daughter Juliana), improving his family relationships and feeling great.

When you opt to look in the mirror, you're going to see the weight. And I'm not just talking about the weight you're carrying on your body. You'll see the emotional weight you carry in your head that makes you eat way beyond what you know is acceptable.

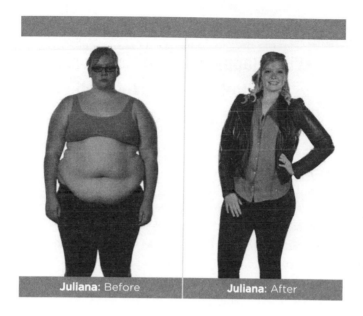

Juliana: Before | Juliana: After

And the weight of responsibilities that make you choose others over yourself. Then there's the weight of your family and friends and the pressure you feel (real or not) to take care of everyone, plus the weight of the tears you've been holding back for years because you have to be strong. There's the weight, too, of shaming thoughts that make you punish yourself with food.

"Weight" has so many meanings. I want you to turn the word "weight" into "wait." "Wait" before you beat yourself up for overeating. "Wait" before you choose someone else over yourself. But *don't* "wait" any longer to change. Do it now. *That* waiting is over.

|||||||||||||||||||||||||||||||||||||||||||||||||||||||||||||||||||||||||||||

What Happens When You Come Face-to-Face with Yourself in the Mirror?

JD,

It amazes me every day how great I feel. The things I am doing now I haven't done in decades. I enjoy cooking with my wife, stairs are not my enemy anymore, and I have to find things to do and not just sit and watch TV. I love working in the yard and finding ways to stay active. Just next Sunday, I am running a Super-Bowl 5K with both my daughters and my wife. My oldest daughter has finally caught the workout bug, and she is working on her own transformation. She is reading labels, eating healthy, and working out every day. I remember how hard it was for me running the first 5K during Boot Camp. Now, I am doing it for fun and to have some family time. Now after a workout, I feel great the rest of the day, and my energy is through the roof. Even though my knees sometimes get tender, I now feel that if they don't hurt at least a little, I haven't worked out hard enough.

—Jeff, *Extreme Weight Loss* cast member, via email

CHAPTER 6

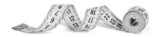

You Are Not Fat because You Love Food—No One's *That* Hungry

Why are you fat? As I described earlier, when I asked that question of our former contestant Stacey, she gave me the stock answer: "I love food." I get that answer nine times out of ten, and it's never the truth. The tenth answer is usually not true either. "I love to cook." "I don't know how to cook." "I can only afford fast food." "I have the fat gene." These are excuses, not reasons, as I mentioned in the introduction. In fact, unless someone starts their answer with "My whole family was killed by a drunk driver" (which someone actually did), I assume they're not telling me the real reason.

So why are you fat? First, let's explore some of the excuses in more depth. *I have the fat gene.* There's no such thing as a single fat gene. There is the "I make bad decisions gene" and the "I was taught bad habits gene," but your family members are fat because of their behavior. You don't have to be like them. Yes, you may have a genetic predisposition that puts you on the chubbier side, but that's no reason to let your weight get completely out of bounds.

It doesn't mean you're doomed to be fat. It just means you have to work harder to keep fit! Coming from the family I come from, I'm living proof of that. And don't tell me that obesity is a disease you're stuck with. Alcoholism is a disease, but do you think alcoholics should still drink? What if they were to tell their families, "I have the alcoholic gene, so it means I'm going to drink. Get used to it"? Drinking is destructive, but so is being so overweight that it jeopardizes your health.

I find it interesting that a 2014 study conducted by researchers at the University of Richmond found that overweight people who read literature stating that obesity is a disease ate more calories than overweight people who were given information specifically stating that obesity is *not* a disease. Of course they did! The way I read this study is, *See, I can't help it if I'm fat, I have a disease, might as well eat what I like.* If somebody gives you an out—whether that somebody is a doctor, a scientist, or yourself—you're going to take it. But whether obesity is a disease or not (I'll leave that to the medical experts), you can't make it an excuse to eat yourself into oblivion.

Other feeble excuses? I've heard thousands of them. "My knee hurts, I can't get on the treadmill." *Excuse.* "My husband won't watch the kids so I can't exercise." *Excuse.* "I'm not a morning person." *Excuse.* "I have two jobs." *Excuse.* "I have to eat what my wife cooks." *Excuse.* "Going out to eat is my social life." *Excuse.* "I work a desk job." *Excuse.* "My dog ate my treadmill." *Impossible!*

These things may interfere with leading a healthy lifestyle, but I'm willing to bet that, whether you're aware of it or not, there is an emotional or psychological issue that is at the root of your weight problem. It doesn't mean that something horrific had to have happened to you. It could be that the stress of life is getting to you and, with poor coping skills, you find solace in french fries. Who doesn't? My weakness is chocolate chip cookies. When I'm having a bad day and walk into the house and smell a fresh batch baking, a cookie is better then sex . . . Okay, maybe not better. But it ain't worse, either!

||||||||||||||||||||||||||||||||||||||||||||||||||||||||||||||||||||||||||||||||||||||||

Read Between Your Own Lines (and Lies), and You'll Find the Truth

Hi JD,

I have to tell you that I have never forgotten the day that I met you, and you asked me to tell you my story because you didn't know anything about me.

For so many years, I have hidden behind the mask of looking like I have it all together, and that day you called me out. Thank you. That was the first time

I even told my story. At that moment, I realized that I was going to change for me. When I put my sh** out there for the first time, and started to have a little pity party, you brought it right back to me and helped me confront that a lot of the things that happened to me, were my choice. Ouch.

I am so glad that I finally let go of every secret, bad choice, failure, and disappointment I have been holding onto for the last 13 years and cried out for your help. For the first time, I am looking forward to my future!

—Charita, *Extreme Weight Loss* cast member,
via email

There could be lots of things boiling beneath the surface. Maybe you're angry, very angry, but have no outlet for that anger. Somewhere along the way, you replaced those feelings with cheesecake and BBQ ribs, and it gave you pleasure. Then, when you kept doing it, your brain took over, associating those foods with feeling good. So now, your brain asks you to repeat the action over and over again. In fact, it's come to the point where the only way you feel pleasure now is to eat those foods.

That mind-body connection is real. Neurobiological researchers have shown that doing something enjoyable, like eating a chocolate cupcake, causes the brain to release a chemical called dopamine. Expose your brain to that hit of dopamine over and over again, and it's going to develop a habit. Your brain is going to make your body crave that dopamine in a gotta-have-it kind of way.

Maybe, though, you have something else going on. Maybe, like Georgeanna, you succeeded at being a great mom and failed to take care of yourself. It could be something deeper, too. Maybe you've never gotten over the pain of parental neglect or the ending of a relationship. Big, small, somewhere in between—whatever it is, you have to deal with it if you want to lose weight. Again, it goes back to what's in your heart and head. Figure out what's eating you, and the pounds will melt off.

It's also possible that your real reason for being fat is locked so deep in your subconscious that you're not even aware of what's holding you back. That means you're going to have to do a deep dive into your life, really look closely, and pick apart, calorie by calorie, bad decision by bad decision, how you got where you are today. Think about the last time you were happy with yourself and work forward from there. Something happened. Somewhere along the way, you stopped being important to yourself. You gave up. The renowned psychotherapist Carl Jung famously said, "Until you make the unconscious conscious, it will direct your life, and you will call it fate." For overweight people, fate is "I love food." "I love to cook." "I don't know how to cook." "I can only afford fast food." "I have the fat gene." And all those other excuses that provide solace because they make it seem like you're powerless to avoid being fat. But there's something else there. You know it, and I know it.

So how do you make the unconscious conscious? Talk about it to anyone who will listen! Attack the situation as thoroughly as you attack a pepperoni pizza! Dig down deep to find the answer to the question: Why am I fat? The other day, I heard a woman being interviewed on the radio who had lost a job opportunity because of her weight. Most people would have dug in their heels and said, "They need to accept me for the way I am." But she was in the performing arts, and she had to face up to the cold hard fact that the performing arts world doesn't work that way. So she made a concerted effort to slim down. In the interview I heard, she began talking about how she got to be fat in the first place. "Food was my best friend," she said.

Immediately, I thought to myself, *Here we go, she's going to talk about how she was fat because she loved food.* But the woman surprised me. She went on to say that while she had had a gastric bypass, it was only a tool to help her get the weight off and that her lack of self-esteem and her self-criticism did not go away when the weight did. She acknowledged that her emotional difficulties had to be dealt with, or the pounds would have come back on. In that respect, she told the interviewer, losing weight was not as easy as she thought it would be. But by addressing the fact that she didn't feel comfortable in her own skin, she was ultimately able to keep the weight off. The weight-loss surgery helped, but she owed her success to confronting her personal issues.

There's no one explanation for why people get dangerously or even just uncomfortably fat, and maybe you already know your (real) reason. Sometimes, though, it takes serious digging to get at the issue (or issues) behind the pounds. Maybe you'll even need a therapist to help you. Don't be afraid to reach out to one. But start the process with some introspection. Make the effort to fearlessly confront and work through the problem. Ask your friends and family, too. Sometimes, they have the insight you need—they've just always been too afraid to share it. But it can help you.

As the woman I heard on the radio discovered, introspection is no walk in the park. People think weight loss is hard because food is tempting and exercise is painful. That's not what's hard. You can do all the exercise and diet stuff. What's hard is looking at your life. But it's the solution. When you start admitting what's really going on, change happens. Yes, that's right. The real work is done in the mirror!

5 REASONS YOU MIGHT BE FAT

1) You have no coping skills.

As I got to know Elaine, the woman I mentioned in Chapter 1 who wanted to lose weight so that she could climb up to the fortress at Masada, I learned more about how she ended up carrying an extra hundred pounds. It wasn't like she was a fat kid; in fact, she didn't start gaining weight until she was in her late twenties and went through a divorce. Some people have the life skills to move on. Elaine didn't. So without the benefit of a supportive family to walk her through the steps of dealing with emotional turmoil, she ran away, landing in probably the worst place for someone in need of comfort: a cruise ship. "It was a great place to disappear," she says. It was also a great place to get fat. For five years, while working on the ship, Elaine did what most people do for only a vacation: She dove right into the all-you-can-eat-and-drink cruise ship culture. And it wasn't even fun. The heavier she got, the more she stayed isolated in her cabin. "I didn't want to feel anything. I was eating and drinking to push down my feelings," says Elaine.

You know how parents teach babies to self-soothe so they don't need to be held all the time? Parents should also teach their older kids how to self-soothe without self-destructively stuffing themselves. Most of us never get taught healthy coping skills, so when stuff happens, we're all vulnerable to the pull of hedonism. When that hedonism gets out of control, it's like a double-whammy. Without good coping skills, an upheaval will send you into the arms of your neighborhood baker, then because you, once again, are lacking coping skills, the shame and embarrassment of cleaning out the bakery will make you continue your descent into overeating. It's a vicious cycle.

2) You're hiding.

Fat is insulation in every sense of the word. Psychologically, it insulates you against painful emotions. Physically, it gives you a place to hide away from the world. Nobody wants to deal with the fat person; nobody is going to come on to you in an unwanted sexual way. People might not even befriend or be polite to you. A man will go the extra mile and hold a door open for a thin, beautiful woman. But for a 300-pound woman? Ignored. And she feels that. "People don't notice you when you're fat; they look through you," says Elaine. Perhaps you like it that way? Mitzi—who you might remember from Chapter 1 as the woman who so enjoyed finally being able to go to an amusement park—did.

When Mitzi began the weight-loss process, she took the time to look at old photographs of herself. The changes—and their causes—became obvious. "I was a normal-size baby, but when I was five years old, my parents divorced and, almost instantly, you can see me going from a normal-size child to getting a little

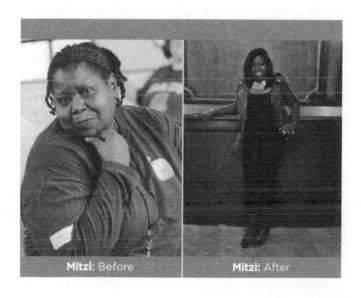

Mitzi: Before   Mitzi: After

chubby," she says. "When I reflect back at different times in my life that my weight went up, each time involved a loss of some sort. My mother and father's divorce, a bad relationship, losing my mother. Getting into my teen years and into my twenties, it was getting attention from older men. If I gained more weight, then they'd leave me alone. It was a way of shutting people out, of not wanting people to be attracted to me in any form or fashion." Instead of figuring out a way to deal with unwanted attention from men, Mitzi, like hundreds of other women, found it was easier to just get fat, ensuring that most men wouldn't even bother.

Elaine saw her weight that way, too. Over the years, she ended up yo-yoing back and forth between fat and slim. Early on in this roller-coaster ride, she realized that being thin scared her. "When I would lose weight, I'd feel emotionally naked," she says. "Fat was like two arms around me, comforting me."

3) You're punishing yourself.

Maybe you see food as a reward. Something you get to indulge in for taking all the crap that comes your way or maybe even for something good you've done. But I see it as a punishment, a form of self-sabotage. You think you don't deserve to be fit and healthy. You're not worth anything so why not drown yourself in a bucket of fried chicken or a huge hero sandwich? For Amber, the realization that she was punishing herself with food was liberating. "I used to always think of food as a positive thing. I like to eat, I don't have a boyfriend—which I didn't back then—I have food. It was a source of comfort and I used it in so many ways. To celebrate, when I was ashamed, everything," she says. "Now I see how I used it as a weapon against myself. That shift was huge."

4) You're trying to fill a gaping hole.

Food fills you up in more ways than one. Or, should I say, people use it to fill a hole; that doesn't necessarily mean it works. In fact, it doesn't. You can eat until the end of time and not fill the emptiness that comes from loss, anger, depression, or loneliness. So many of the overeaters I've met were stuffing themselves because they had lost a parent or because a romantic relationship had gone south. Loss and emptiness in life translates to a feeling of emptiness in the stomach. You'd think that exercisers were, on the contrary, doing the healthy thing. But this same transference can be found among extreme exercisers. You can run a hundred miles and still be sad and lonely—and crazy in my opinion. I would ask that person, "What are you running *from*?"

5) You are more stressed than you know.

To my mind, there are two types of stress. There's the everyday stress that you can't help but be all too aware of. *I'm late for work. I'm not making enough money. The traffic makes me crazy. My schedule is too packed. My kids aren't doing well in school. My parents lean on me too much.* And so on. Then, there's the other kind of stress, the cause of which hasn't bubbled to the surface. You don't know what's going on, but something is, because you can't stop eating. You might even think you're perfectly happy—you love your boyfriend, you love your job, you have a good relationship with your parents, your glass is half-full. But there is also a little bit of a nagging feeling in the far reaches of your mind, and of course the unhealthy living. What explains that?

Scientists have a name for people who manage not to consciously experience stress: They're called repressors. Maybe you're one of them. If someone asks you how things are going, you say, "Great!"—and really mean it, even though your body and behavior tells a different story. In one 1997 study, published in the *Journal of Personality and Social Psychology*, researchers asked people to give a speech to a small audience. Some of the speech-givers, who were identified before the study began as repressors, said they were not nervous about speaking—but their heart rate numbers gave them away: Their hearts were fluttering just as fast as the hearts of people who reported being very anxious about the speech. It wasn't that they were lying either. They just didn't realize they were anxious about the speech.

I know that, in my own life, I'm not always clued in to stressors going on beneath the surface. In the 20-plus years that I've been married, my wife and I have never had an argument that wasn't about something else. "What are you upset about?" she'll ask me. "It can't be because the kids didn't put their books away." And she's right. It never is. I am usually upset about something else—maybe I'm even upset at myself about something—but I don't always have the ability to verbalize or even understand what it is. My wife, on the other hand, understands how to diagnose me before I am even conscious that there is a problem. Which is why I love her.

You'll be taking a big step in the right direction if you stop thinking about what things seem like on the surface. "I love food too much." "I have no willpower." That's not it. No one is going to know what's inside of you, so you have to figure it out. Let other people help you. Talk things out. Have someone close to you ask you leading questions. The more exploration and, yes, the more crying you do, the closer you'll get to discovering the issue you need to deal with. That's how the weight will come off. It's not about counting calories.

PART II

Make a List of Things You Need to Do

CHAPTER 7

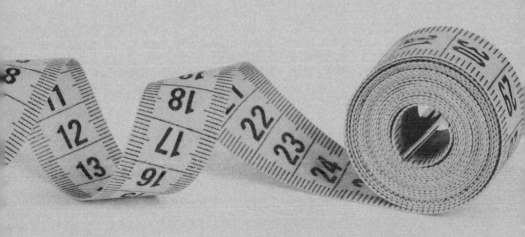

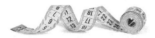

Be a Contestant on Your Own Reality Show

Maybe (I hope!) you've been watching the weight-loss shows I've created over the past 12 years, all the while thinking to yourself (perhaps with a pint of Häagen-Dazs perched on your lap), "I could do that, too, if I just had *The Biggest Loser* Ranch or *Extreme Weight Loss* Boot Camp, the trainers, the refrigerators full of healthy food, the camaraderie. If I had all that, of course I could be skinny!" But what if I told you it wasn't the Ranch or Boot Camp or the trainers or the food or the friendships or even me yelling at them that has led all those cast members you've watched cut their body size in half? What if I told you that the key transformation that leads to their success happens way before they even step into one of our gyms? In fact, it happens before they even make it on the show.

What is this magic ingredient? I am sure you'd like me to sprinkle that pixie dust on you! Well, I can. The process that potential cast members go through *before* they even get on the show has a huge impact on how well they do. That process involves filling out a questionnaire and making a video of themselves, which sounds simple, but it's not. What it really involves is asking how they got to where they are and how committed they are to change. And to spark our interest, they can't just give superficial answers to our questions. They have to dig down deep for the truth and display a real understanding of themselves. And let's just say that we're looking for those people who are pulling out the backhoe, not the garden spade. Don't assume that's because we're just interested in lurid stories that will play well on TV. What we're interested in are people who are going to lose weight. (I have always said that if we had contestants with great stories but they didn't lose any weight, we would be off the air in a matter of weeks.) We know that, in order to do that, they have to come face-to-face with what got them to a reality-show tryout in the first place. If in that video and questionnaire they can (finally) be honest about why they're fat, reveal what's going on beneath the surface, and stop putting a pretty face on their troubles, they are on their way to success. We constantly ask them to dive deeper, and we give them feedback to lead them in the right direction.

In fact, no matter what comes back on the questionnaire and video, we always tell them to dig deeper. We give them tips like, "Ask your kids how they feel about having an overweight mom/dad. Ask your co-workers, too. Ask your spouse if he/she is still attracted to you." We put them in dangerous emotional positions to see if they are committed enough to go there. If they shy away from these interactions, we know they are not ready. On the flip side, when they lean in, ask the hard questions, and get emotional in the process, we know that they are moving in the right direction toward transformation. While I can't personally give you feedback, you can get it from the people in your life. You just have to be brave enough to ask the right questions. It's part of your "precasting" process.

What the precasting process will do for you, too, is help convince you that you can do it. By the time our cast members meet the trainers, they're already convinced; there's pretty much no stopping them. It's like a tree in the forest that has been hit by an axe 30 times. All you have to do to get it to fall over is blow. The Ranch, Boot Camp, trainers, nutritionists—all that stuff is just puffs of air pushing along something that's already about to happen.

I believe that the precasting process can help *anyone* get a jumpstart on weight loss and transformation. But you have to take it seriously. Treat it like your job. Remember, the root of transformation is DESIRE!! So here's what you're going to do:

- Answer the questions beginning on page 96. These are identical to some of the same questions we ask potential cast members. Don't just read them and answer them in your head. Get on your computer or take out several pieces of paper and a pen, then give detailed answers. If it doesn't take you a couple of hours to complete them, you're doing it wrong. Go deep. Some answers might take you a couple of days to process. Let it all sink in; really think. Even talk about it with friends, co-workers, even your mother (who may have helped make you fat in the first place). Talking about it will start the wheels turning and give some clarity to thoughts you have been struggling with for years.

- Videotape yourself telling me why you should be on one of my shows. Choose someone you feel comfortable with to hold the camera, or shoot it yourself. Either way, be prepared to open up. Don't say to yourself, "I would never humiliate myself on TV just to lose weight, so I'm not going to humiliate myself on videotape either." Swallow your pride, and just do it. Interview friends and family, too. Ask them what they think the source of your problem may be. You'll be surprised to learn how willing your family and friends are to be honest when there's a camera on them.

They'll tell you what they see and, more important, what they wish for you. All of their answers will be clues to help you determine how to be happy. If you are not finding yourself uncomfortable, and maybe even in a flop sweat while doing this, you ain't doin' it right!

Playing the role of a contestant will help you immensely. These tools will give you incredible insight into your own pain and the issues you need to deal with. They'll help you formulate your own personal to-do list and a plan to put those to-dos into action. But only if you really go for it! Be insanely diligent about going through the process. While you can do this on your own, I like the idea of enlisting someone to help you. You could even have a friend interview you using the questions that follow. As you'll see as you read on, you're going to need to start talking to other people about your goals and progress. Start now!!

Start the Truth-Telling Now: Here Are 20 Questions to Help

1. Is weight an issue in the family you grew up in? Who suffers from it? How much weight do they need to lose? Do you blame your family for making you overweight?

2. What is your ethnicity? Does your culture play a part in your weight?

3. Describe your occupation. Does your weight affect your occupation? How?

4. What's it like being overweight? How does it affect you in your everyday life? How exhausting is it?

5. What are all the things you missed out on being at this weight?

6. What activities are difficult at this weight, either physically or emotionally? List anything from getting in and out of cars to getting undressed in the locker room at your gym without feeling self-conscious.

7. Does weight interfere with your life as a single person, person in a relationship, married person, or parent?

8. What would it mean to you to be at a healthy weight?

9. Have you ever been thin? Why haven't you lost the weight?

10. How did you gain the weight?

11. Describe your diet from the minute you wake up to the minute you go to sleep.

12. Food to me is _____.

13. Do you have kids? Have you passed on your poor eating habits?

14. Are you afraid of dying prematurely due to your weight?

15. Describe how your family upbringing has played a part in your weight gain.

16. Have you let yourself down by being overweight? Have you let your family down by being overweight?

17. What do you see when you look in the mirror?

18. Is there anything about you that you haven't even told your significant other or your best friend?

19. How much weight do you want to lose?

20. What is going to be different this time around?

Again, really answer these questions thoroughly. Don't give one-word answers because you think no one is going to read them.

Imagine you are desperately trying to get on one of our shows, and you know the answers to these questions could make or break your chances. The answers *matter*. The very act of writing may bring issues from your subconscious into your conscious so that you become fully aware of the reasons you've been unable to lose weight in the past. Your "sickness" (overeating) is an emotional illness. Figure out the moment of emotional impact that's driven you to lose control and you'll never need to go on a diet again.

Let me say it again. I am looking for you to pinpoint the exact moment or moments in your life when you began to view food as a source of comfort, rather than as fuel to feed your body. Once you identify this, you start your transformation. This moment (or moments) might seem like a small thing—perhaps someone called you ugly, or you had a fight with your mother—but for you it was a major issue and you are still feeling the repercussions.

By going on the same journey as the cast members on our show, you are effectively becoming the Sherlock Holmes of your weight issues. This detective work will be a big wake-up call. All those issues that have been swirling around in the back of your mind for a long time will come to the forefront, ready for you to deal with them head-on. So use this information to good purpose. Look at it again and again as you go through the weight-loss process to remind yourself why you're doing this—and why there's no going back.

I want to mention one thing that you should also be on the lookout for during this process of self-examination. You may actually find that you're not ready to do this yet. You may have thought you were, but you're not. It happens. Let me tell you one cautionary tale. We had a guy named Wally try out for *The Biggest Loser*, but he turned out to be too big for the show. Imagine that. Too big for a show about fat people. I felt so bad sending this guy home to a most certain future of sickness and early death. Maybe, I thought, there is a way we could help people like him, too! So my business partner, Todd, a guy named Adam Greener, and I came up with an idea for another show—the show that eventually became *Extreme Weight Loss*—that would help people who were too big to be on *The Biggest Loser*. We called them the super obese.

To pitch the show to ABC executives, we screened a video of Wally struggling to put on his socks. That was literally the whole tape. It took him 5 minutes to get just two socks on his feet. As he struggled to do something we all take for granted, I saw the show buyer tear up. We walked out of the room with a deal. In a sense, Wally made it happen for us; the executives were hooked on the idea of seeing that super obese man (and others like him) fix their lives on TV.

When we told Wally, he was thrilled. "That's amazing," he said. "You guys are going to change my life."

"Okay, just send us all your paperwork so we can get started," I told him.

Weeks went by and I kept calling, trying to get him to send us his questionnaire and other information. "It's in the mail," he'd say.

"Send it," I'd say, "or I'm going to fly to Chicago and get it myself. I want to help you, Wally."

Finally, the paperwork came in, but only after I called, emailed, and threatened to show up at his front door. The show started filming. For the first 90 days, Wally did well. In fact, everything was going better than we had all hoped. Then his wife called. She couldn't find him; he'd been missing for 24 hours. We went to the house to keep watch for him to come home and eventually he did—with a car of nearly 20 (we counted) fast food wrappers. Ultimately, we helped Wally check into an in-patient weight loss facility. He just wasn't going to be able to do it with our help alone.

The moral of the story is that, while you may feel (and act) gung-ho at first, you're not ready if you cannot do the interior work it takes to change your life. That was Wally's downfall. The fact that we more or less had to drag him to the starting line should have alerted us to that fact. That was a live-and-learn moment for us. You will have to be the judge of whether you are prepared for the challenges that lie ahead. If you are just answering yes or no to the questions I asked you on pages 96–97, it's a sign that you don't yet have what it takes to succeed. (Which doesn't mean you won't be ready sometime down the line!) But if you're ready to go deep, then you're ready get on with it and ready for success. The weight is going to fall off—just watch.

CHAPTER 8

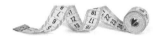

Break Down and You'll Break Through

The first thing I learned on the very first season of *The Biggest Loser* was that fat people want to talk about their feelings. The problem was, in their normal lives, no one had cared enough to ask them to share what was going on in their heads. They not only received no encouragement but they felt invisible—even though they were the largest people in the room. It was as if everything they were experiencing didn't matter.

I got a pretty rude awakening during the first interview we did with a *Biggest Loser* contestant. Suddenly, a grown man was crying. Not just crying. Blubbering. At first, we all stood there not knowing what to do. But we quickly learned that the man's crying (and the crying of many of the other contestants that would follow) was the sign of a phenomenon we'd see again and again: After a breakdown, an incredible breakthrough followed. When anyone finally let out what had been bottled up inside for years, the pounds fell off them with the greatest of ease. The discovery was monumental: **Tears weigh more than fat.**

Throughout the years, getting people to talk about what they're feeling has proven to be a formula for success. We've seen cast members go from dropping zero pounds in a week to having an emotional moment—opening up in a way that they never have before—and, as if by some miracle, achieving double-digit weight loss the following week. This hasn't just happened a few times; it's happened dozens of times! What is so powerful about unlocking the subconscious and letting the tears fall that helps people who have always failed at weight loss start succeeding? I'm no shrink (in fact, there are times that I think I could benefit from one!), but I can confidently say that it's because tears weigh more than fat. As I've been saying all along, fat is just a symptom of something bigger. You are not fat because you love food. Just acknowledging that something lies beneath starts the ball rolling—and it's all downhill from there.

I'd say that 90 percent of the people we cast on our shows come on thinking that they're just going to deal with their eating and exercise habits. If only that were all they needed to do! That would be a walk in the park. A lot of them will try to get around digging below the surface, but we force the issue. And, eventually, they get it: Diet and exercise and the process of dealing with emotional baggage go hand-in-hand—and feed on each other. Jennifer, who you might remember had lived a trauma-filled life, saw the connection early on. "The more weight I lost," she says, "the more I was able to say good-bye to my past." Yet in the beginning, she was terrified. Most people are. But it's the only way out. Fear, sadness, secrets—they weigh you down. But once you address their origins, you'll be lighter in every way.

Earlier, I told you a little bit about Bruce. He's the young guy—28 when he came on *Extreme Weight Loss*—who was wary about losing that jolly fat-guy persona, something his friends loved about him. Believe me, that was the least of his problems. One day, when Bruce was in ninth grade, he came home and there were police cars everywhere. His father was being arrested on 22 counts of sexual molestation, but Bruce didn't understand why until he read an article in the newspaper (and it was front page news): Several kids from his Pee Wee football team had come forward and accused Bruce's father of molesting them. Bruce had never even heard the term sexual molestation—and he didn't understand that what his father had been doing to *him* since he was a young boy was also sexual molestation. He thought his father was his best friend. To him, it was normal—that's what your father did. Bruce's mother worked the night shift and left the house every night thinking she was leaving her son in a safe place.

After Bruce's father went to jail, the kid ballooned north of 400 pounds. "I was just fighting to survive in my life, battling to keep a roof on our house and food on the table. I didn't worry about what I looked like," he says now. "Plus, I just thought I was fat because I loved to eat food. I didn't want to face the real reason why. I didn't want to use what had happened as an excuse. Poor me. So many other people use drugs; my drug was food." At the heart of it all, Bruce was still battling with the notion that he had never been truly loved by his father. He realized that what his dad wanted from him was wrong—but even from prison, his dad still had an emotional hold on him. And it was choking Bruce to death.

When we first met, Bruce was leading a seemingly normal life, working as a high-school football coach and inspiring his players with his go-for-the-gusto personality. But he still hadn't dealt with the past. Whenever there were hearings at the board of pardons, he'd go and try and connect with his dad—and, as unbelievable as it sounds, advocate for him to get out of prison. I asked him, "Why would you try to connect with someone who did unspeakable things to you and other kids? Why wouldn't you try to keep him in prison for the rest of his life?"

In his final sit-down with me during the finalist selection process, Bruce's hands shook and his eyes released the biggest tears I have ever seen. Then he said something I still struggle to understand. "My dad was the best dad ever," he said. "We did everything together. We were inseparable." With a body now more than 400 pounds—clearly a sign that something had gone seriously wrong in his life—Bruce had still not come to terms with the fact that his dad never loved him in an appropriate way. Yet even with all the abuse that man handed out, he could not put out the inner light inside this kid. Bruce was broken, for sure, and he wasn't even aware of how broken he was. Still, his spirit endured.

Bruce had originally tried out for *The Biggest Loser,* and I did not pick him. He seemed so out of touch with the truth, and unwilling to deal with the pain in a way that would help him transform. Undaunted, he kept coming back year after year, trying to get on one of our shows. Each time he came back, I heard a new version of what he wanted from life, and slowly I started to believe that this kid could scale any wall to success.

What helped swing the pendulum in his direction was the fact that Bruce started to lose weight on his own. He lost 50 pounds *before* his final audition. Even before I told him he had officially made it onto the show, I had a private meeting with him and let him know that I was the only one who thought he could do it— and that I don't like looking like a fool. I asked him point blank, "Are you going to let me down?" He didn't even hesitate and said, "I am going to be your greatest success ever. Let's do this thing!"

Call it luck, call it coincidence, but the season he finally made it onto *Extreme Weight Loss,* his father came up for his final parole hearing. If he didn't get released then, he'd have to serve out his life sentence.

By the time of the hearing, Bruce had lost a lot of weight (he ultimately lost 185 pounds) and, more important, gained confidence. He'd spent considerable time working with a therapist and dealing with what had happened to him. He'd also proved to himself that he could get a handle on his eating and transform his body—he was "the man" now in so many ways. Still, from day one, Bruce was adamant that he didn't want to go to his dad's hearing. I told him I would honor his wishes, but that he should really think about how powerful it would be to look his dad in the face as a new man, and let his dad know that he no longer had any power over him.

Bruce and I spent a lot of time talking about how he could close that chapter in his life and make sure that his father would never hurt him or any other kid again. Bruce had been carrying a lot of guilt about his silence during the years of molestation; now was his chance to speak up. Finally, just a few days before the hearing, he decided to go—and our cameras went with him since the hearing occurred during the filming of Bruce's episode. As you can imagine, for Bruce, walking into that board of pardons hearing was like walking into hell. Several members of his family were there arguing *for* his father's release, so speaking out *against* his dad—who never once turned around to look at Bruce and even denied under oath that he abused Bruce—took considerable courage. Yet he spoke forcefully and swayed the judge, who said she didn't believe Bruce's father's denials of abuse. His father is still in prison and, because Bruce was so courageous, will be there the rest of his life. The weight finally came off Bruce and you know, of course, that I'm not talking about body fat.

Bruce is one of the most inspiring guys you'll ever meet—so inspiring that we hired him as a trainer. He now works for *Extreme Weight Loss*. In the 12 years that I've been doing weight-loss shows, I'd never hired a cast member to train anyone before! That's how special he is. I often tell his story when I speak to groups because it just shows you what can happen when you tackle the mind-sets, the head trips, the subconscious twists and turns that contribute to being overweight. During the weight-loss process, Bruce became his own man. Does he still have darkness? Yes. A lot. Is he still fragile? Very. But he took steps to improve his life. And continues to take them every day—it doesn't just end once you lose the weight. Just as you have to adopt healthy diet and exercise habits for a lifetime, you have to stay on top of the psychological and emotional reasons you put on pounds.

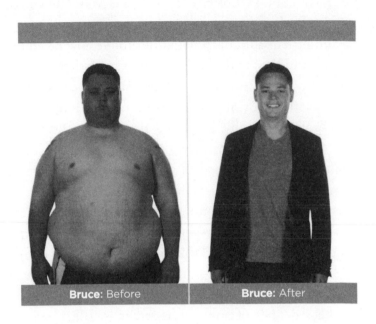

Bruce: Before   **Bruce**: After

What it boils down to is attitude. One of my favorite sayings from Bruce is, **"The only thing in life that's not hereditary is your attitude."** Any psychologist will tell you: You can't always control what happens to you in life, but you can control how you interpret and react to the crappy hand you're dealt. That is 100 percent up to you. Of course, it's hard. And I'm not just telling you to put on a happy face and everything will be all right. But keep in mind who you want to be and adopt the attitude of that person. *Be the person you know you are deep down inside.*

Here's a story about someone who did exactly that. One thing I haven't yet told you about Mitzi is that her problems extended beyond being overweight. Mitzi, 52 when she joined *Extreme Weight Loss*, doesn't like the word *hoarder*, and rightly so, if that brings to mind a slovenly person. Mitzi, in truth, is a lovely, well-put-together woman and no one had a neater room during Boot Camp. Nonetheless, things had piled up in her house to an alarming degree. A better way to put it might be to say that she could have been on an episode of *Extreme Hoarders*. And nobody knew. She had kept it a complete secret, telling friends from out of town who wanted to stay with her that she was going to be away. She'd never invite local friends over, either, and when anybody did drop by, she'd pretend she wasn't home ("It was so strange, your car was in the driveway but you didn't answer the door"). Not one friend had been to her home.

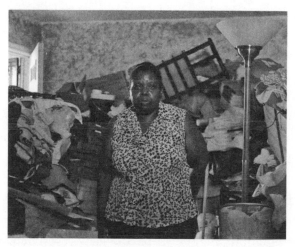

Mitzi in her house

What feelings Mitzi could not push down with food, she pushed up against her front door so no one could get in. Emotionally, you could not get into her head, and, physically, she shut everyone out with the mountain of objects piled up high in her house. So for Mitzi, confronting the issues in her life didn't just mean dealing with what was leading her to overeat and resist exercise, it meant facing up to what was making her live in chaos. Add to that the fact that she would be doing so in front of millions of television viewers, and, naturally, she was fearful. "My body was cluttered and my life was cluttered, and the thought of opening up that aspect of myself to reveal the whole Pandora's box of my life was terrifying to me," says Mitzi. Most people come on our show to overcome one addiction. Mitzi would have to overcome two!

Mitzi had actually gotten on the show by happenstance. She accompanied a friend who was trying out for the show and we ended up encouraging her (not the friend) to go through Boot Camp. But though she'd signed on, she was ambivalent and even tried to quit the show, emailing staff members and thanking us for the opportunity but acknowledging that she just couldn't do it. We eventually talked her down. Emailing back, I pointedly told her three things: Don't let the *situation* stop you. Don't let *fear* stop you. Don't let *you* stop you.

Mitzi didn't respond to my email right away. Instead, she told me later, she called a friend. They talked for three hours, and Mitzi told her about the hoarding; it was the first person she'd ever told about the problem (we knew about it because we'd been to her home as part of the casting process). What a *huge* step to tell someone! The first step to healing.

Mitzi's friend reminded her of a joke that I think is relevant to anyone who's hesitating on opening up his or her emotional life in order to bring about change. It particularly resonated with Mitzi, who's a very spiritual person. It goes like this:

> A town is flooded by rain. A man escapes his home and stands on the rooftop. A boat comes by and the driver shouts out, "Get in, let us help you."
>
> "No," says the man, "I'm waiting on the Lord." Next, a helicopter hovers above him. "Grab onto the rope," the pilot yells.
>
> "No," says the man once again, "I'm waiting on the Lord." One after another people come to help the man

get off the rooftop, and each time, he turns them down. The water rises and the man drowns.

In Heaven, he meets God. "Lord, I was waiting for you to save me. What happened?"

And God says, "I sent a boat, I sent a helicopter. . . ."

Could you be doing the same thing? Certain signs may be there. Say your doctor told you that you have to give up frozen yogurt with ten candy toppings and hop onto a spinning bike, or else. That's a sign you get. But the signs that you also need to attend to are the emotional reasons behind your weight gain; signs that, out of fear, you may be missing. Like Mitzi. Her friend laughed at her. "Mitzi, do you realize that God's been sending you a sign the whole time? You accompany a friend to a casting call, and out of 6,000 people, you get picked for a show you weren't even trying out for?" If that's not a sign, I don't know what is.

Mitzi and Bruce are extreme examples of people keeping their real feelings inside. Their problems were monumental. Most of you (I hope) aren't going to be dealing with sexual abuse and hoarding, but that doesn't mean you don't have to start talking about what's going on. Maybe the problem is that you hate your job, and your boss is an jerk. Quit and work somewhere else? You can't. You need that medical insurance, which your spouse doesn't have, and you have a mortgage to pay. So, every day you go in, and you're miserable. The only time you feel good is when you open that drawer in your desk—and I've heard this story a bunch—and that bag of M&Ms is there. For a moment you feel free. Or maybe it's your marriage. You can't get divorced; you'll end up broke or without your kids. You feel helpless.

The gravity of your problem isn't really relevant to what I'm trying to say because this goes for everyone: Figure it out, and deal with it. You've picked up this book; that means you want to make a change. So don't say now's not a good time. There's never a good time for drama, so most people tend to push the real reason they're fat down further and further from their conscious thought. And I get it. You're so busy going to work, getting the dry cleaning, picking up the kids, doing your volunteer work, making food for the big family dinner at your sister's house, there's no way you can stop and say to your husband or best friend that there's something that's really bothering you and start opening up. There isn't time for it. How do you wake up one day and declare, "I'm going to do this emotional work on my own during the ten minutes I have between my shower and making my kids breakfast?"

I know one thing that works for sure: **Me . . . confronting you.** Not letting you off the hook with your standard BS line about why you're overweight. Of course, I'm not there to challenge you in person, to climb inside your head and play mental Ping-Pong like I do with the people on our shows. This is not guesswork. It works every single time. I have 12 years of proof. Nonetheless, imagine that I *am* there testing you, pushing you, backing you into a corner, and making you shadowbox out of it. If that's beyond your power of imagination, find someone who won't let you off the hook. Instead of walking through life in a dark room unable to see the truth that will heal you, I need you do to whatever it takes to start turning the lights on.

Maybe it's a friend, or maybe you need to get professional help. On our shows, we have the luxury of pairing people up with therapists, something that may or may not work for you. But, okay, say a therapist is not for you; it's not your only recourse. Just get started in some way. When I made Stacey go home and tell her husband about the secret she'd been keeping from him, it opened the floodgates. Do you think she would have done that on her own? No way. She had already spent 20 years hiding it, why bring it up now? It took a metaphorical smack in the face for her to realize that it wasn't impossible after all. And after she did, her whole life improved. In every category, life got better, but she had to confront her biggest fear first. That blind leap of faith is easy to write about, maybe even easy to consider for someone other than yourself. But the reality is, if you don't bring yourself to do it, emotional recovery is not possible.

However you handle it, here's the bottom line: Stop pushing the problem away. Let it bubble to the surface. Acknowledge it. Then take a step. From where I'm sitting now, the door is 75 feet away. I can't reach the door in one step; it would be impossible no matter how far I can jump. But as long as I take one step—it doesn't even have to be a big step—I will be closer to the door than I was a second ago. If I stay in my chair, I'm definitely not getting closer to the door. Get out of the chair; that's the first step. You don't have to climb a mountain. You just need to take one step. And remember that view out that door gets better and better as you get closer to it.

CHAPTER 9

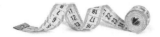

Keep Your Promises

I already keep my promises! I can hear you saying that to yourself under your breath. How could I even think that you don't keep your promises? Relax; I know you keep your promises—your promises to everyone else. You probably keep promises to people you barely even know. Well, how about keeping a promise to yourself for a change?

I get it. When no one is watching, it's easy to break a promise to oneself. But when you tell your sister you'll watch her kids on a Saturday night, that's a harder vow to break. There's going to be some blowback on that one. That keeps you honest. I bet you're the best friend, worker, family member anyone could ever have. You'll promise virtually anything, and then you'll always deliver. You'll pick up your friend at the airport in rush-hour traffic, no problem. You'll do the extra two hours of work because your boss wants to go home. You'll go to your brother's house and feed the cat. You'll do it all, just as you said you would. Yet when you say to yourself, "I promise not to eat that doughnut," your word of honor goes out the window in an instant. It's so easy to keep promises to everyone else and sacrifice yourself in the process of doing it, but can you keep a promise to yourself? If you're reading this book, you've broken a promise or two to yourself, whether it's to eat right or to go to the gym or to address the emotional turmoil you're holding inside.

Some of the best promise-keepers are soccer moms and dads. Maybe this will sound familiar. You pour yourself into doing things for your kids. *I promise to pick you up from school and get you to the field on time. I promise to spend the whole weekend traveling to and from tournaments. I promise to get you to your tutor, your music lessons, your community service.* While you're making good on all these promises to your kids, the pledge you made to yourself to stop eating chips in the car in between dropping off the fifth grader and picking up the high-school junior falls by the wayside. The vow to work out on the treadmill for an hour every morning gets broken as quickly as it gets made. And I get it. I'm devoted to my kids, too, but there has to be balance in family life or, ultimately, no one comes out ahead. And remember, using those reasons as a way to explain why you didn't stick to your promise to yourself falls under the category of *excuses*!

It also goes back to what I asked before: What are you teaching your kids by eating chips in the car or not going to the gym? If it's okay for Mom and Dad to hit the snooze button, it's okay for me to do it, too! But if your kids wake up at 6:00 a.m. to a note that says, "I'm in the garage riding my stationary bike, get ready for school, I'll take you when I'm done," you've just taught them a lesson about healthy living without them even knowing it. Wow! Your kids won't listen to a word you say, but they watch every move you make. That mental imprint is something they will have forever. So help them make a positive impact that will pay dividends to their future.

Of course, it's not only people with busy family lives that break promises to themselves. There's the single woman who promises to go out for hot-fudge sundaes with a friend crying over a breakup—sending her own vow not to eat ice cream down the drain. And the

THE BIG FAT TRUTH

recent college grad who promises to watch the game, drink beer, and eat pizza with the guys—even though he's sworn off beer and pizza. Once again, promises to others, kept—promises to oneself, broken.

||||||||||||||||||||||||||||||||||||||||||||||||||||||||||||||||||||||||||||||

The Best Surprise Is When You Surprise Yourself

Happy Thursday!!!!!

I'm ba-a-a-a-a-ack! Finally back in L.A. and I started my day at CrossFit and then a hike with some of the crew!

I still can't believe Monday's weigh-in—I lost 6 pounds on freakin' vacation! Who does that?!? This girl! Finally living a life of no excuses and true transformation!

Thanks for all your undying support!

—Cheyanne, *Fat Chance* cast member, via email

In my 12 years as a producer of weight-loss TV, I probably never met anyone who sacrificed themselves for the sake of others as much as Raymond and Robert, whose generosity toward their family knew no bounds. These identical twins have been the backbone of their family since they were 12 years old. It was then, while they were living with their three sisters, their father long gone, that their drug-addicted mother first went to jail. For the next few years, while she cycled in and out of prison, the boys got the other kids (including their older sibling) up every morning, bathed, dressed, and off to school, all the while hiding their parent-free existence from social services. "We knew that if we went to school every day, no one would think twice about us," says Raymond. So they did, and they did well. These kids were savvy enough to know that if their grades were good, the teachers would never ask to speak with their parents. The fear that social services would come in and split the kids up into multiple foster homes was enough for the twins, at age 12, to become the heads of their household.

At first, their grandmother tried to help them, but after she went through two bankruptcies trying to support them on her salary as a cashier at Wal-Mart, Raymond and Robert started mowing lawns after school and taking other under-the-table odd jobs on the weekends to buy groceries for the family. Just a houseful of kids with no parent in sight! It's inconceivable to me how two 12-year olds could figure out how many lawns to mow in order to put food on the table, but somehow they kept doing it. And in a way, they still were when I met them at age 26. Working without pause for 14 years—most recently at a windows and doors manufacturing company—they were still helping to support the family. One of them had even become a supervisor.

Health-wise, though, they were a mess. The social stress of hiding the fact that their mom was in jail, trying to keep the kids together, scheming to earn money for food, and having to be adults at such a young an age took its toll emotionally and, by extension, physically. They were so busy worrying about everyone else (and working so hard to pay for everything, including the babies their sisters had without other means of support), that they pushed their own needs to the side. "At a younger age, we were athletic and played sports so we didn't think the fact that we were a little bigger than everyone else was any big deal; we were in shape," says Raymond. "But once we graduated, we just got bigger and bigger. I got up to 450 pounds by the time I was 21, and Robert was 422."

I ask you, would it be bad for the brothers to turn their attention to themselves for a while? Two guys who had been through everything, including homelessness and sleeping in their car? Of course not. Fortunately, they finally did decide to do something to better their own lives, and what happened in the lead-up to joining the cast of *Extreme Weight Loss* simply amazed them. To attend Boot Camp, the twins would need to stop working for 90 days. Given the financial impact, three months off could have been a deal-breaker, but the family banded together and agreed to pay Raymond and Robert's bills while they were away. The twins couldn't believe that, for the first time in their lives, the tables had turned—somebody was actually going to help *them*. Had they never taken action to help themselves (by trying out for *Extreme Weight Loss*), they would have never even known that kind of help was an option. That was their blind-faith moment. When they finally sought help, it brought the family even closer.

I think you, too, might be surprised that all those people you've been helping might like the opportunity to help you for a change. Not everybody, naturally, but in my view, people are more generous than you might ever imagine. Before anyone can promise to help you, however, you need to make a promise to yourself that you are going to get healthy, mentally and physically, then keep that promise as if your life depended on it (because it likely does).

Sometimes—make that often—keeping promises to oneself means being self-centered. That might go against every instinct you have, but it's necessary, at least for a while. *You* are your priority right now. If you feel that you can't do that, take a page from Mitzi's playbook.

Mitzi, as you might remember, actually got on *Extreme Weight Loss* by accident when she accompanied a friend who was trying out. The staff encouraged her to fill out the paperwork, so she did; next thing she knew, she was in Colorado for a week of finals casting. At one point, Mitzi packed her bags, thanked everyone, and asked to go home. But we saw something in her, and we wanted her to stay. I personally spoke to her about continuing on and joining the show. Mitzi works for a nonprofit that helps homeless families living in transitional homes and domestic violence shelters. Every day of her life is selfless, so it was hard for Mitzi to take the time to work on her own problems. "Mitzi," I asked, sitting down next to her and looking her right in the eye, "don't you believe that you deserve this? You deserve just as much as what you give to others. You have the golden ticket, and you deserve it and so much more. You deserve to be loved. You deserve to live in a safe home." I promised her we would deal with her issues respectfully. She was still not ready to say yes. I told her to go back to her hotel and sleep on it.

Several "aha" moments followed. For one thing, the old airline mantra—"Put on your own oxygen mask before you help others" started to run through her head. "I always felt I had a purpose in life and that purpose was to help others help themselves," says Mitzi. "But I really felt that I couldn't do it to full capacity if I wasn't helping myself. I kept thinking back to the oxygen mask metaphor." Yes! You will be a better worker, friend, sibling, child, parent, member of society if you are a healthy, happy person. Even if you are the ultimate promise-keeper and humanitarian, you will be even *better* at it when you take care of yourself.

So that was one lightbulb that went off in Mitzi's head. The other one was this: It was time to start practicing what she was preaching. "I had been teaching the children I work with to be okay with who they are and to let their emotions be out there, yet I wasn't applying that advice to myself." She was acting like life was superfantastic when that was far from the case.

Keeping your promises to yourself means being authentic. It also means not cutting corners. If you say you're going to work out for an hour, don't work out for 59 minutes. Because the next thing you know, 59 minutes will become 58 minutes, then 57. You get the picture. There are no shortcuts. And don't let anyone else take them when it concerns your well-being. Don't let your spouse toss your salad with the cheesy Caesar dressing because it's easier than putting your portion in a separate bowl before tossing. Don't let a trainer let *you* show up late for your workouts. If she's letting you get away with stuff, she's not the right trainer for you. Be an advocate for yourself. And, by the way, if a trainer is not a good fit, try another one. Keep trying until you hit gold! When you go shopping for that perfect outfit, do you try one on and quit? No! You might try on dozens before one feels right, so why would you not do the same thing with your life?

Even the most minor of promises like, "I promise to do laundry today," needs to get done! If you put it on the list, you have to get it done. In my house, we have a saying we live by: "Do what you have to do before you do what you want to do." I tell my kids if you *want* to watch TV, do the homework you *have to* turn in tomorrow first. Putting things off, or only doing 80 percent of something never leads to success. And the resulting feelings of failure can be toxic. Shame creeps in with the potential to put you into a downward spiral. So instead, make those promises to yourself, and do what you have to do. Say it out loud to yourself as you are taking off your shoes and kicking your feet up on the couch instead of going for a walk. **Do what you have to do before you do what you want to do.** It will train your brain to prioritize and help you get the important things done—like exercise—before you're too tired to do them. You want to go home and hang out with your roommates or family? Fine, but first do what you have to do—that is, go to the gym.

Approach promise-keeping just as you would any other aspect of weight loss—one step at a time. Don't take on a giant promise—"I'm going to eat only fruits, vegetables, and white meat chicken from now on" or "I'm going to ride my bike 20 miles every morning"—on day one. And don't make 20 promises at once. It's too overwhelming. Just make one small promise—"I'm going to pack my lunch today instead of going to the Thai place with my work friends"—and keep it. Keep it for a week. It will feel good. Add another promise. Keep it for another week. It will feel even better. Build on all your victories, and each successive promise you make will be easier to keep.

Honoring promises you make about exercise and eating right is going to feed into other areas of your life. Those continuing education classes you promised yourself you were going to take so you can get that promotion at work? You're going to finally enroll. The vow you made to stop letting your sister take advantage of you? This time you're saying no. Breaking up with a boyfriend, telling a girlfriend it's over? Done. Looking better naked in the mirror is great, but the real goal here is to improve your life.

CHAPTER 10

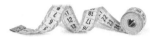

Stop Being a Puppet—Pull the Strings of Your Own Life

There's a famous guy I know who trains Special Forces, the military unit that performs dangerous and unconventional missions. In one of his classes, to use combat as a metaphor for life, he takes 20 guys and lines up 10 on one side of an imaginary line, 10 on the other, facing one another. Then he puts a bag of ice and a rag next to each of the first 10 men. To the 10 guys on the other side of the room, he says, "I'm going to count backward from 10 and when I get to zero, you lean over and hit the guy across from you as hard in the face as you possibly can. Knock him out cold." Crazy, right?

Now the guys that are about to hit someone don't know if he's serious. If he is, they're thinking that if they don't throw the punch, they're probably going to get kicked out. Meanwhile, across the room, the other guys are freaking out because they're about to get punched in the face for absolutely no reason. As the instructor's count gets down to 2, and sweat is literally dripping from the potential aggressors' faces, he stops and asks, "What's wrong? Are you guys nervous? You don't want to hit someone in the face?" And, of course, they start saying things like, "I don't even know the guy. I don't want to hit him."

Then the instructor says, "Okay, great. Everyone with the ice and the rag, move it to the man across from you. I'm going to count backward from 10, and when I get to zero, you lean over and hit the guy across from you as hard in the face as you possibly can. Knock him out cold." The situation is now reversed. They were going to get punched in the face, but now they're the aggressors. They're the ones allowed to throw a punch, and they're excited about it. Why? Because a minute ago they were going to be the victim, the person not in control of what was about to happen to them. Two scary words here: "victim" and "control." Which is better? To wallow in being a victim or to get mad and do something about it—to take control?

Who's the Boss of You? You!

Struggling today. Wanted a Diet Coke, but resisted. Held a cookie in my hand today for Emma (she had an end-of-soccer-season party). Thought about biting it but didn't because that cookie isn't worth the pain I have been enduring. Emma offered me a piece the size of a very small crumb. She said that I could only have a tiny piece because cookies have a lot sugar (she's five). Had a great workout this a.m. in my yard with my girl Peggy. This afternoon I burned about 500 calories raking leaves. Learning to exercise when stressed instead of eating.

—Christina, posted on *The Revolution* Facebook page

The instructor never actually lets the men hit each other. He is just trying to get across this message: Is it better in life to get hit or to be the one throwing the punches? Don't take this too literally.

I'm not telling you to go out there and start acting like a jerk. What I *am* telling you is to take control of your life. If you've been getting metaphorically punched in the face for years, maybe it's actually starting to feel good. Think back to what I said about failure being your happy place. I think there are other happy places—and that you'll find them if you just put yourself in charge of your own life.

Your mission now is to start being the puppeteer, not the puppet. Being in control of your life is powerful. It's sexy. It's exciting, especially if you've felt out of control for ages. I say "felt" because don't tell me that you don't have control over your life, because you do. *I can't help it.* I hear that cop-out every day, and I'm not sympathetic. Many people—and many overweight people especially—genuinely believe that they are not in control of *any* aspect of their lives. They can't control what happens to them at work, how much money they make, how their family treats them, and, above all, they can't control what they eat.

I don't buy it. In fact, I think it's complete BS, because everyone has a choice. You can choose a better way. You have power that you have not yet put to work. Fear is in the way. Remove the fear, and amazing things start to happen.

Trina, a woman we had on one of the shows, was a perfect example. Trina was a grown woman, in her forties, a nurse, married with two kids. And yet her mother ruled her life as if Trina was still a fourth grader. Her mother would drop in at Trina's any time she wanted, showing up sometimes at 11:00 p.m. to do her laundry. Did she call first? No. Of course, she didn't call first. And her mom was mean, too. "What makes you think they'll pick you for the show?" she said to Trina. "They'll never pick you." What do you think Trina did every time her mother finally went home? If you said, pull out the carton of ice cream, you're right.

"Trina," I told her, "you have to create some boundaries, set some rules."

"But she's my mother!" Trina would argue. "I can't do that."

||||||||||||||||||||||||||||||||||||||||||||||||||||||||||||||||||||||||

Ask and You Shall Receive

So today we are at the mountain, right, and I'm driving myself crazy because every time I go there, I have a tradition of enjoying a hot chocolate and sitting in the cold air by the outdoor firepit and enjoying the beautiful view. I finally decide I'm just gonna go ask the hot chocolate girl if she has anything that I can drink. (I don't drink coffee.) I told her I was on a mission to lose weight. She was so nice and went out of her way to start pulling out packages and reading labels and what not.

Anyway, guess what? I got to have my moment by the fireplace! She made me a "Vanilla Steamer." It was a cup of nonfat milk: vanilla-flavored, sweetened with Splenda, and cinnamon. OMGosh, it was so good. And I didn't feel guilty.

So, the point is . . . don't be afraid to ask people to help you. Sometimes, they are more than willing to do it.

—Shannon, posted on *The Revolution* Facebook page

"Okay, Trina, then you will always be 300 pounds and unhappy. Your lack of boundaries is bad for you, bad for your marriage, bad for your kids, and bad for your family as a whole. What person in her forties is still at the mercy of her mom? What husband would even allow that?"

It took months of cajoling, but finally Trina read her mother the riot act. She set boundaries for when her mom could come to the house, and she changed the lock and didn't give her a key. And what do you think happened? Her mother actually listened to her—and Trina started losing weight in a big way.

Knowing that you can make a decision and stick with it is empowering. You don't have to start taking control of everything tomorrow; I've seen people start taking control in small ways, then work their way up to being the puppeteer in much more consequential ways. Say, for instance, that you go out to dinner with your spouse, who orders dessert for the two of you. You can sit there and dig in, all the while listening to your inner voice shame you for doing so. But what if you cut the dessert in half and say, "Honey, here's yours," take one bite of your own portion, open up the salt shaker and pour salt on top. It's drastic (and, okay, a little gross), but it's taking control of your environment. You can no longer say, "I can't help it, dessert was thrust upon me." Own it! Be proud that you took control. Even brag about it. Again, it's all about the brain game. Your subconscious is not aware you used salt to destroy the dessert. All it knows is that you kept your promise not to eat it. Do that a few hundred more times and you win.

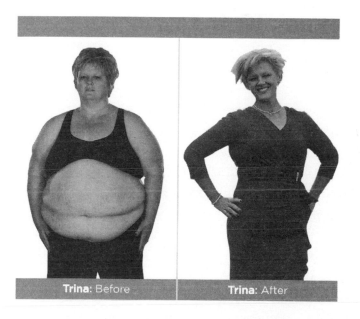

Trina: Before   Trina: After

Look, I know it's hard to have restraint. For instance, there is no way that anyone can sit with a package of Oreos in front of him and eat just one. It's impossible. I can't even do it. They're scientifically engineered to make you want more, and you can't beat science. If you eat one cookie, you're going to have another one. Maybe you don't even like Oreos, but I guarantee that there's something out there that's your Oreo.

But, once again, wrestle that temptation to the ground. If you want an Oreo, go get one. Go the vending machine, buy the little package of cookies for $1.25, open it, eat one, then dump the rest in the garbage or give them to someone else. This might sound like a minor act of resistance, but it will make you feel powerful and in control. Being in control is like a having a super power.

I know what you're thinking: "That's so wasteful." And not living up to your potential isn't? Which is the bigger waste? One package of $1.25 Oreos or not living a full life? Don't start about starving kids in Africa—that's another problem entirely, which eating more than your share of sugary foods is not going to solve. In the long run, wasting food at these moments is a better option than endangering your health.

You're going to find that when you begin to assert yourself some of the things you thought were impossible to control really aren't that difficult. One of the things that made it difficult for Raymond to have a healthy lifestyle was his work hours. Raymond worked the night shift and slept during the day, a schedule that he said was not conducive to working out (*excuse!*). But after he got back from Boot Camp, he pressed for better hours—and he got them. Why? Because his bosses valued him more than he had previously valued himself. When he finally put his foot down and said, "I work days, or I need to find a new job," they realized they couldn't lose him. Alert! This was after going through Boot Camp for three months, where he was taught to place a high value on his well-being. He put the work into himself *first*, then starting demanding better in his life. And he earned it. Don't just wake up tomorrow and demand things. Earn the right to demand better.

The lesson here is that, when both Raymond and Trina at long last laid out the boundaries that worked for them, both boss and Mom agreed to the terms. So ask yourself, are you, like Raymond and Trina were, selling yourself short? If you don't hold yourself in high value, how do you expect other people to?

Sometimes, you can feel so beaten down by failure and people saying "no" that you give up asking. Don't. Get out there and start asking for the changes you need to support the lifestyle you desire. You won't always get exactly what you want, but the point is you need to find out. Don't admit defeat before you even know what you're up against.

When you start feeding your emotional and psychological needs rather than your stomach needs, the universe has a crazy way of correcting all the wrongs. Work hard, get healthy, and make good choices, and rewards usually follow. But the number-one thing you need to focus on is consistency. Show up to the gym every day no matter how you feel. Eat the right foods even when you want to cheat. Repeat these "good" behaviors until they just become "normal" behaviors. Be a robot. Get your mind and body following one message: Today we get stronger, smarter, fitter, healthier! Repeat and repeat and repeat.

CHAPTER 11

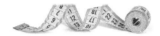

Shout It from the Rooftops

People are always worried that they'll be embarrassed if they tell others that they're trying to lose weight. Guess what? They already know that you're fat. Not only is there no shame in admitting you're trying to slim down but it's *imperative* that you tell people. In fact, the more people you tell, the more likely you are to succeed. Silence will be your downfall; speaking out about what you're doing is your insurance policy. It's your pixie dust.

Let me explain. One thing I hear all the time is, "Yeah, of course, you have a great success rate on your shows—the cast gets trainers and nutritionists and all kinds of people to help them, something the average person cannot do." True. But I also know lots of people who hire trainers and nutritionists and all kinds of people to help them, and they still don't make a success of it. What our cast members have that works better than all the diet and fitness experts in the world is millions of people watching them. That's the pixie dust, the magic potion that makes the pounds disappear. Nobody wants to fail while millions of people are watching. The television cameras keep our shows' participants honest (the opportunity to win $250,000 on *The Biggest Loser* doesn't hurt either).

So how do you replicate the all-eyes-on-you experience of a

reality contestant? You create your own pixie dust at home by making sure you have an audience. Post your pictures and intentions on Facebook. If you're really brave, you'll get a shirt made that says "I'm going to lose 100 pounds this year" and invite people to ask you about it. Talk about it to anyone who will listen. If that's too public, call a select group of friends and family to tell them, or join (or start) a weight-loss support group. Consider approaching someone in the gym who looks like he or she might be a good mentor. It doesn't matter how you get the word out. Just let what you're doing be known.

There are two reasons for this. One is accountability. Knowing that there are people watching how much you're eating, how much you're exercising, and how many pounds are dropping off you makes it much harder to cheat, to quit, or to fail. The people you tell are going to check in on you, and you have to give them the right answer ("Yep, no dessert this week, 60 minutes on the treadmill every day"). I always know when one of our contestants has fallen off the wagon if they're no longer posting pictures of themselves on Facebook. Once you go public, you can't hide, even if it seems like you can. And it works. Statistics from 75 million users of the online weight-loss tool MyFitnessTool show that people lose three times as much weight when they share their food diary with friends. Use examples like this to play the odds and increase your chances for success!

The second reason for shouting your goals from the rooftops is pride. It's embarrassing to admit that you can't do something that you said you could. When you take on the job of changing your life, it's like standing on a cliff. A television camera watching makes it a very high cliff—you're not going to want to jump off your new habits; it's too dangerous. But when you're doing it all alone, and nobody is watching, that cliff is a lot closer to the ground. It's no big deal to jump off. So don't do it alone. Spread the word about what you're doing, and it will be as effective as living your life on live TV.

|||||||||||||||||||||||||||||||||||||||||||||||||||||||||||||||||||||||||||||||||||||||||

Here's What Happens When You Enlist Someone to Check Up on You . . .

Hey JD,

Okay, so I had just gotten home and had decided to put my hike off until tomorrow (like I tend to do these days), and my phone pinged with an email . . . um, it was from you, and I kid you not, I jumped up right then and put my tennis shoes on, loaded my dog up, and went!

Thank you thank you thank you for checking in on me because I feel *great*—although I was huffing and puffing on that hike! I wouldn't have gone if I hadn't gotten your email! I feel proud and, of course, I don't want to let you down. Zumba tomorrow morning at 9:30 a.m.!

—Ashley, *The Biggest Loser* contestant, via email

The next day, I heard from Ashley again . . .

Hey JD,

So got up this morning and went to my first Zumba class! [She sent me a picture to prove it.] Wow! Kicked my ass, but I made it, and it felt good. I went to the car when it was over and almost left without buying more classes, but I got out and went back in and bought a card, so now I have to go back! Still fighting that voice saying, "that's too hard, you can't do it." So far negative voice 0, pink ninja 2!

—Ashley, via email

As you probably know, we have thousands of people who try out for our shows, and some of them keep coming back year after year. (Bruce, for instance, tried out for *The Biggest Loser* seven times and *Extreme Weight Loss* twice before making it onto the show.) I always wonder why, if they want it so badly, they don't go home and do it on their own? You really don't need cameras to succeed. One of our cast members, for instance, beat out almost six thousand people for a spot on *Extreme Weight Loss* only to then get cut from the show. Since she had made it to the finals, she did get to go through the first week of Boot Camp. To her credit, she took the knowledge she gained during those eight days of nutrition and diet education, went home and lost 50 pounds on her own without any cameras (or trainers or diet specialists pushing her to succeed) before getting a call back. A little bit of knowledge—and telling many of the people in your life that you've committed to a goal—can go a long way.

Sadly, though, most people leave their auditions, go home, and live life as they always have. We had one guy who tried to get on the show three years in a row. The third year, he made it to finals week, and we really liked him. He owned a pizza shop and was a real character, but he couldn't pass the medical exam. He did get to go to Boot Camp for a week and learn all about what he needed to do to lose weight. But he was angry about not getting on the show, and it defeated all the good he was starting to achieve. He went home and decided not to put all the information he'd gathered to work. Three months later, at age 50, he died of a heart attack. I felt bad that he fell through the cracks, but I also can't help but wonder what would have happened if after that first year of trying out for the show, he went home and lost the weight on his own. Would he still be alive today? Would his daughter have a father to walk her down the aisle? Would his wife have grown old with the husband she loved? Chances are, yes. What could have been fills me with sadness.

So what are some ways that you can go about working "cameras"—that is, other people—into your weight-loss plan? First, figure out what kind of support is going to work best for you. You can zero in on a few people or tell the world via whatever social media platform you use. Post a "before" picture of yourself on Facebook. It might not be millions who'll see you make a promise, but even if it's only 50 people, you have, in effect, scattered the pixie dust. To avoid embarrassment, you have to keep going. And I guarantee you are inspiring others. Remember when I talked about the best backup plan being no backup plan? This is the same thing. You will have one choice, and one choice only. Don't play it safe and say, "Oh, I am not that kind of person who can do this publicly." Get out of your comfort zone. Take a risk. Don't be afraid of embarrassment or losing friends; be afraid of living lies and half truths.

If you're telling just those special few, think about who's going to hold you accountable in the most effective way. Find someone who knows how to push the right buttons for you. If you respond best to gentle encouragement, get people that you know will be kind but firm on board (if, however, they're going to give you a pass, and act all sympathetic when you pig out at a party, you're relying on the wrong pals). If you know yourself to be best motivated by the drill-sergeant type, get your best no-BS friends and relatives to be your go-to people.

Stay open to anyone who offers help. You may find that you actually need a different kind of mentoring than you think you do. I remember one of *The Biggest Loser* contestants told me that she needed a soft touch to help her lose weight so, of our two top trainers, she wanted to work with Bob Harper. I gave her Jillian, maybe the least gentle trainer on Earth. Yet the contestant actually responded really well to Jillian's tough-love approach, probably better than she would have to the Zen-like Bob. She didn't know it was possible, but tough love brought out the best in her.

What's really critical is finding someone who believes in you, not just someone who can offer advice or accountability. Find someone you don't want to disappoint. To be honest, I think a lot of our shows' participants stay on track because they don't want to let me down. I remember one, in particular, who worked very hard not to disappoint me. Initially, everyone on the casting team except me voted to drop him from the pool of potential candidates. I argued for him and, eventually, we put him on the show (being the boss has its advantages). But I didn't let this little bit of behind-the-scenes maneuvering go unnoticed. I told him point blank that nobody wanted him on the show, including the network, but that I owned the production company, and I was choosing him. My neck was on the line; if he failed, I failed. Sounds cruel, but I happened to know that this was the exact button to push. And it turned out I was right. This was not a guy who liked to disappoint anyone.

He was elated not just because he made it into the cast, but because, finally, somebody believed in him. Someone fought for him and took a risk on his behalf. Later, when I saw him on the field going through a brutal workout, he yelled out to me, "You've just made the best damn investment in your life!"

"I know I did," I called back. That cast member was Bruce.

There's another element to this shout-it-from-the-rooftops thing. Tell people what you're doing; get the inspiration of all eyes on you in place. But also ask people for help. It's a must. You have to do it. It's very, very hard to lose weight without help. Ask someone to literally check in with you a few times a week to see how you're doing. Ask a friend who is a paragon of dietary virtue for some food ideas. Maybe he or she will even give you a cooking class. Find people who have already lost weight and kept it off, and ask them for advice and even to be your mentor. People who've been through it want to help you—they know how good you're going to feel when you totally make over your life. If it's someone you don't know but have seen at the gym, get the story. How did she do it (people love to talk about the ins and outs of how they lost weight)? Would he be willing to be an accountability partner or mentor? You are asking for people's time, which is big, bigger probably than asking for people's money. But I can assure you that there are multiple people out there that will be happy to give it. It will surprise you.

A lot of our cast members have been blown away by how supportive family and friends turned out to be. While she was in Boot Camp, Amber's mom got up at 4:30 every morning to walk Amber's dog three miles, then her stepdad would ride his bike with the dog along for another three (if only Amber had been working out as much as her dog!). Her mom would then exercise with a personal trainer for an hour (whom she hired after being inspired by her daughter's efforts), drive the dog back to Amber's house, go to work, then drop back by the house to pick up the dog again. She did all that for the three months Amber was in Boot Camp. Amber's mom also helped get her daughter's house in order so she could create a gym in the garage and be ready to cook healthy meals when she returned from Boot Camp. Now, that's love.

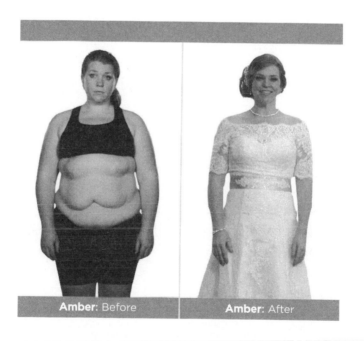

Amber: Before   Amber: After

One reason I speak so passionately about depending on other people to help reinforce your healthy lifestyle habits is that I do it myself. I know what I'm not good at, and one of those things is running alone. I am a runner, and I love it. For the last 20 years, I've run 30 to 35 miles a week. But I can count the number of times I've run alone in the past 10 years on one hand. I don't like to run alone. Okay, I hate it. Each mile feels like 10, but when I run with my guys, each 10 miles feels like one. So I took control over it by organizing a running group. Everyone shows up at my house at 5:30 a.m., and we go. Notice I said that we meet at my house. That means I have to go. Imagine if I just decided to bag it. These guys would be banging at my door at 5:30 a.m. without hesitation!

The group has been together for more than ten years and has evolved. People in the neighborhood know us as "the guys that are always running." It has become not only my social time with these friends but something more. It's crazy how you will open up to a guy on a ten-mile run, telling him things you would never tell anyone else. That's why I'm such a big advocate of workout buddies. It not only keeps you accountable, it can provide you with a particular and very special kind of friendship. Now not only do the members of my running group help each other stay fit but we meet for dinners and breakfasts and read a book together every year. It is social time that doesn't require an unhealthy intake of alcohol, chicken wings, and fried cheese sticks, but serves the same gratifying purpose.

This is something you can do. It doesn't have to be a running group. It could be a walking group or a share-healthy-recipes group. Anything. One thing you have to get over if you're going to do this thing right is any shyness you might have. I know—you don't want to be a burden to anyone. Asking for help isn't your style. Make it your style. Put yourself out there, and be vulnerable; people will respond. And membership, as they say, has its privileges. In this case, it's the privilege of staying accountable and, maybe, if you're lucky, making an incredible connection with someone else.

I swear by the buddy system because of my own experience and because I've seen how integral camaraderie is to our cast members' success. But don't take my word for it: There is plenty of science to back it up. Just recently, researchers in the Department of Preventive Medicine at Northwestern University took a look at how much of an influence "friending" had on people signed up for an online weight-loss program. The number of friends a person had in the website's online community was directly proportional to the amount of weight he or she lost. Users who did not connect with others lost about five percent of their body weight over six months, and those with a few friends—two to nine—lost almost seven percent. The social butterflies (those with more than ten friends), however, lost more than eight percent.

||||||||||||||||||||||||||||||||||||||||||||||||||||||||||||||||||||||||||||||||||

Like-Minded People Will Rock Your World

JD,

The 400-meter run was difficult for me today. Bruce Pitcher, who is my mentor, did the lunges with me and then said, "Let's go, Rod!" as we chug-jogged out the door. But before I got to the door, Brandi jogged next to me, and then AJ jogged next to Bruce, and Sara jogged next to Brandi, and as we jogged out the door, Mandy jogged behind me. Josh was finishing his last 400, turned around and jogged with us, then Cassie turned and jogged again.

We were all jogging. Together. Like a team. . . . Those guys had all done their workouts already. That last 400 meters for me? That's another shining example of what this is and has been for me. It's been about the relationships and the connections, about the love. I just felt it in the biggest way. And that is everything.

—Rod, *Extreme Weight Loss* cast member, via email

Joining an online community is a great way to go, but there are plenty of ways to establish community. Think about other ways you can draw people into your cause. Get their (and your) competitive juices flowing. Ask your boss to put up a $50 Whole Foods (or healthy market near you) gift certificate for a three-month challenge: see how much weight, percentage-wise, everyone in the office can lose. It drives conversation—and it drives you. Instead of, "Morning, what did you binge watch last night?" it becomes "Did you work out last night?" What you're doing is building a community of like minded people who are there to help each other (you included!) stay in step.

CHAPTER 12

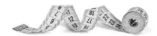

Stay Out of the Crack House

You just posted your goals and your picture on Facebook. You called friends and told them you're going to lose weight. You announced it at a family dinner. You've told everyone the news and gathered all these people around you. Now figure out who should stay, and who should go. What do I mean by that? Some people are going to lift you up, support, and inspire you. Other people are going to drag you back down to where they like you—stuck in the sedentary, face-stuffing, miserable old days where they still dwell.

And if you think you can weather the influence of friends and family, I'd ask you to think again. In 2007, researchers at Harvard Medical School and the University of California, San Diego who analyzed data from over 12,000 people found that a person's risk of becoming obese was 45 percent higher if he or she had a friend who was obese than it would be otherwise. Even if a friend of a friend is obese, the risk rises 25 percent. Have a friend of a friend of a friend who is obese? Your risk rises 10 percent. It extends to family, too. If an adult sibling became obese, your risk increased by 40 percent; if a spouse became obese, your risk rises to 37 percent. Fatness is contagious.

This is brutal, but it has to be said: Many of your friends and family members will not want you to succeed. If you don't want to go out for tacos and pizza anymore, whom are they going to eat with? Your wanting to live a better life puts them in (what they see as) a terrible position. There's the real possibility, too, that your success will make them feel worse about the way they neglect their own health. You're fixing yourself, but they haven't even set foot in the repair shop.

You'd think that the people who love you the most would be your biggest cheerleaders. They'll be so happy for your success! Um, most likely not. It's a bitter pill to swallow, but most people prefer to have others around them that validate their way of life. When you make major changes, that validation goes away. Hopefully, your friends and family will surprise you, but don't take it for granted that you will feel supported by all the people who supported you in your old way of life. It may happen, but you can't count on it. What I've seen time and again is that the people you think are going to support you are the very ones that don't. On the other hand, you'll be surprised by some others who *do* support you. They will come from places you didn't expect.

Approach the situation warily. Just like alcoholics, you have to have people around you who are "in the program." Recovering alcoholics don't work in a bar. So think about how your friends and family have aided and abetted your eat-a-thons and fast-food way of life. (In some cases, it may have been part of the reason they were with you in the first place. You could always be depended on to go out for drinks and chicken wings.) Remember Panda, the guy I introduced you to in Chapter 2 who always felt too weak to lose weight? During *Extreme Weight Loss* Boot Camp, we sent Panda home to talk to his parents about some of the things that had happened during his youth. It was a revelation in more ways than one. "Going home, I realized that a lot of my memories with my friends are all tied in with food," he recalls. "I was driving around the city, saying, 'Oh, my God, there's that restaurant we'd go to, there's the best doughnut shop.' I could see that those relationships that revolved around food were either going to have to go away or change."

That realization didn't make it any easier. "People don't like change," says Panda. "Oh, what do you mean you can't go to lunch with me . . . you're too good for me?" When you change, even if you don't say it, you're implying that your former partners in crime need to change, too. That can cause a lot of friction, which is unfortunate because seeing someone you love do something monumental—and it's no joke, when you consider how many people fail at it, losing weight is monumental—should inspire, not demoralize you.

||||||||||||||||||||||||||||||||||||||||||||||||||||||||||||||||||||||||||

The Power of Love

Hi JD,

I love what you said about how important it is to have someone hug you, be told that you are loved, and have someone really believe in you. I truly found that with [my fitness trainer] Steven. It has made all the difference in the world to me. I walked into the gym with a lot of self-hate, shame, and a hard heart. How much I have changed as a woman. It has been a total gift to me to be encouraged, pushed, and loved (and, of course, having fun while doing it!!).

—Elaine, via email

Part of the weight-loss process for Panda—as it should be for you—is drawing up the strength to say no. In the beginning, Panda found he'd always break to someone else's will. Even if he was trying to eat healthfully and he went to, say, a BBQ or a fried chicken place, he would ultimately indulge. I mean, come on! Who goes to McDonald's and orders a salad? If I want salad, I'll go to a salad place. Places that sell fatty ribs soaked in sauce and chicken deep-fried in oil are not the places to go if you want to eat healthfully. You have to avoid restaurants that might kick off a food memory and make you pick something you know isn't going to be good for you. That may mean avoiding the people who stubbornly cling to your old haunts—they don't want to go anywhere else. For Panda, that meant letting the promise he made to himself override the inclination to give his friends a good time.

Again, you have to look at overeating and inactivity as you would a drug addiction. Who do people who are hooked on drugs hang out with? Other drug addicts. If they get off drugs, then go back to hanging out with the same group of fellow addicts, what happens? They end up back on the drugs. You have to get rid of those friends and start over—which is painful for everybody—or you need to hope that those people can make adjustments. If you don't insulate and protect yourself, it's so easy to fall back into the same old ways. Meet people at a bar . . . you drink. Meet people at a gym . . . you work out. Do the math. Think of it this way: It's time to choose you. Tell anyone not being supportive that it's time to join you, or that you won't be hanging out with them. Like I tell my kids: You are whom you stand next to. If you stand next to people who don't take care of themselves, guess what? It won't be long until you are adopting similar behaviors.

During the talks I give to cast members of *The Biggest Loser* and *Extreme Weight Loss,* I repeatedly warn them about how their relationships may suffer when they leave Boot Camp and go home. This isn't me going all doomsday on them; it's just that I've seen friends and family undo someone's hard work too many times. When I sound the friends and family alarm for the cast, though, most of them react badly to the news. "It's my best friend; of course she wants me to succeed." "Why wouldn't my husband want me in a sexier body?" They may and they may not, but if they don't, it's not because they don't love you. We've had people whose parents didn't want them to lose weight because they didn't want them to feel confident enough to leave home. We've had mates—husbands, wives, girlfriends, boyfriends—who've felt the same way. They think that if their significant other gets thin, they'll leave them.

And sometimes they're right. But people don't leave because they've become thin. They leave because they've become happy, and they want to stay that way. They leave because they weren't really happy before they lost the weight. You don't all of a sudden fall out of love by getting thin; you just realize you want more out of life.

Unless, of course, your mate decides to go on the journey with you. Suddenly, you find him getting up at the crack of dawn to join you for a run, or you find her preparing a healthy, low-fat meal that she learned to cook just for you. Sharing the experience versus having a passive (or, worse, unsupportive) partner makes all the difference in the world. The chances of your relationship making it through this life change go up exponentially if your partner joins in the transformation.

After spending 90 days in Boot Camp, the people who appear on *Extreme Weight Loss* go home on the 91st day with a new way of life and quite possibly a feeling of independence that they never had before. The contestants on *The Biggest Loser* contend with an even bigger disparity since they've been away for a longer time. They go home after six months having lost way north of 100 pounds feeling as though they are different people.

But, as is often the case, everything has changed for them, while nothing has changed for their friends and family. While they spent months looking in the mirror, doing the work of changing inside and out, their loved ones have usually spent months looking out the window, maybe dreaming of change, but not changing a bit. Their husbands are still sitting in the same recliners with the same plates on their bellies watching the same TV show with the same food stains on their T-shirts. Their wives are still cooking the same meals. Their friends are still going out for pizza and beer. Their co-workers are still racing out the door to happy hour as soon as its quitting time. I can't tell you how many people we've had on our shows who, after they lose the weight, go home and quit their jobs or leave their spouses. They realize that they are in a toxic situation—whether it is at work or at home—and that if they hope to maintain all that they've gained (and lost), they have to shake things up. Some people even move to a different state. It's all part of the same trajectory: Change your attitude, change your habits, change your life. Realize that you deserve it. Put value on your own life, and surround yourself with people who share the same value system.

My goal isn't to break up families or friendships. The best-case scenario is one where getting healthy adds a new dimension to your relationship or brings out the caring side of those closest to you. That can happen and it often does. Friends and family that get on board by transforming their own habits seem to get closer to the person who initiated the change. But I can also say I don't regret that we helped some people gain the emotional toughness they needed to walk away from unhealthy relationships. (By the way, many people on our shows have formed healthy relationships with each other and gone on to marry. There are lots of *The Biggest Loser* babies.) If you come home from the gym and your husband is waiting impatiently for you to head out for your usual Friday night ribs and onion rings, that's trouble. He may mean well—he missed you while you were gone and is eager to spend time with you—but he obviously doesn't understand what you're going through. One way or another, that has to change. And more often than not, when you play the card of "you either start supporting me, and better yet, also get healthy yourself, or I am choosing a better life," the other person snaps to attention and learns to get in line. That doesn't necessarily mean he has to come to the gym with you, but it does mean he needs to take care of the kids so you can.

Let's also look at this in a different light. Your decision to clean up your lifestyle provides the perfect opportunity for your family and friends to pull together and become even closer. Lean in and say, "Let's do this together." When someone loses weight and deals with issues right alongside you, it's an act of love, demonstrated through actions, not words. It can trigger the rebirth of a relationship. I've told you about how cast members often go home to find that nothing's changed. Well, there are also times when they go home after months only to discover that their mates spent that whole time losing weight themselves. What better way to show love than to achieve the same goal? It's like saying, "I love you, I love us, and if you can do it, I can, too." When friends and family take up the challenge, it honors you in every way.

Love can be a beautiful thing when it is expressed in a selfless way. Remember the vow "in sickness and in health, till death do us part?" Taking the "health" part seriously can take a relationship to a new level, closer and stronger than it ever was! Reaching new heights in health together opens doors to activities and life experiences you never thought you would share. Now isn't that better than eating a dozen doughnuts for breakfast?

Georgeanna, the wife and mother who devoted herself to her family to the tune of an extra 150 pounds, had great success getting her family on board—her husband, Scott, lost 50 pounds while she was away at Boot Camp. What's interesting about Georgeanna is that she was having an internal struggle about her weight for a long time before she attempted to do anything about it, but she never told her family how bad she was feeling about herself. "I didn't want to burden them," she says. "They weren't aware that I was struggling, and they didn't say anything because they didn't want to hurt me." The lesson here, I think, is that you just have to give people a chance to help you. Don't count them out until they prove that they're not going to offer you the support you need. Georgeanna's family did rise to the occasion, and they helped her by encouraging her and, in her husband's case, losing weight himself.

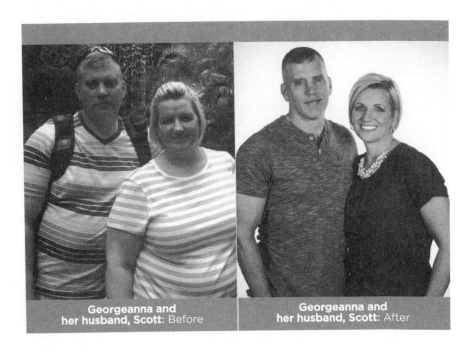

Georgeanna and her husband, Scott: Before

Georgeanna and her husband, Scott: After

On the other hand, if some of the people you love don't see the changes you're making the way you want them to, give it time. Keep doing what you're supposed to be doing, saying no to them when you need to, and most of them will eventually come along for the ride. They'll realize this is the new you. They have to because you're not going to go back. So, they can either get on board or go away. It's hard to take that position, but it's critical. You have to draw a hard line. Give it time, offer your trust, but cut the cord if you have to. I think you'll be surprised to find that, when you ask for more, people are often willing to change.

PART III

Now
Go Do It!

CHAPTER 13

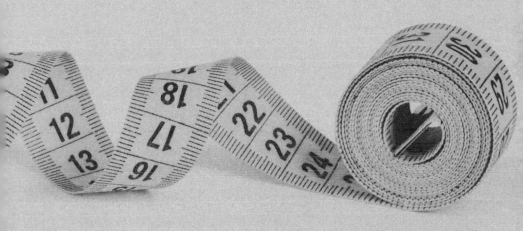

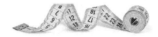

1 Change a Week = 52 Changes a Year

You're now ready for action. So what's the first thing you should do? Dream big, but start small. What you see on TV when you watch *Extreme Weight Loss* or *The Biggest Loser* is what I like to call the nuclear option. It's drastic. Overnight, people go from doing laps around the drive-thru at McDonald's to doing laps around a track and never eating at McDonald's again. They go from having last exercised in the fifth grade to burning 7,000 calories through physical activity in one day. It's a radical approach, but bear in mind these two things: One, most of the people on our shows are pretty much at the point where they need to make up for lost time—illness, if it hasn't already arrived, is knocking at their doors; and two, it's TV. I'm not going to pretend that we don't try to put on a good show. There is inherent drama in the nuclear option that plays well on the small screen. (Although I don't want to give the impression that the people on our shows are nothing more than props to us. No one is more passionately in their corner than us; we are their biggest fans!)

Even without doing something like burning 7,000 calories in

one day, the changes our cast members' bodies go through is nothing if not dramatic. To me, it just proves how strong the human body is. Imagine going for several years, most times decades, doing barely any physical activity, reaching more than 400 pounds, then, all in an instant, stopping all your bad behavior, eating well, and working out four to six hours a day, seven days a week. How can the body withstand such an immediate U-turn? It not only does, it thrives on it. The change is amazing to watch, and results are instant. The body adapts quickly to both bad behavior and good. Fuel your body with good, nutritionally dense food and get your blood moving by exercising, and that engine you have called a heart triggers a metabolic change almost immediately. We have people who come to us with gray skin, no energy, and on multiple medications for life and within 30 days, look younger, have tons of energy, and go off all the medications doctors claimed they would need for the rest of their days.

Any changes you make are going to have an impact, and the more dramatic the change, the more dramatic the impact. Without heavy support from nutritionists, trainers, and doctors, the nuclear option might not be viable for you. But, you don't need the nuclear option to be successful. For the average person, baby steps actually work just as well. The classic approach to weight loss is to change overnight. You go from sitting in your recliner and stuffing down 5,000 calories on Sunday to running the track at the local high school and eating 500 calories on Monday. How long is that going to last? I'll give you until Thursday, tops.

It doesn't even have to be as drastic as that to go bust. I have a friend who cycles through change. "Buddy, from now on I'm only having juice for breakfast, and I'm working out two hours every day." Maybe it doesn't sound that hard, but I know that for him, it is. He'll talk incessantly about all the changes he's going to make, which lets me know that he's only three weeks away from not doing it anymore. Consistency is everything. This guy actually went on a three-day juice cleanse in preparation for a trip to Vegas for a three-day bender that was to include eating and drinking himself into oblivion at the hotel buffet. Why bother if you're not going to follow a cleanse with clean eating? Don't reward good behavior with doing something bad. Nothing drives me crazier than when, after a 60-minute spin class, covered in sweat, someone steps off her bike and says, "Now I can afford that chocolate cake today." *No, you can't!* Reward good behavior (spin class) with good actions (eating well).

Making extreme changes can work, but only if you have a plan for eventually finding a happy medium between all or nothing. Most people don't, including all the people who go on juice cleanses. To me, juice cleanses are mostly moronic because people think they're doing something really good for themselves. You won't have to cleanse if you don't get "dirty" (that is, constantly eat crap) in the first place. If you're just juicing, then going back to your old way of living, well, I don't have to tell you that nothing good will come of it. For this same reason, I'm against diet books that use sleight of hand to make you believe that you can lose weight quickly and keep it off without changing your lifestyle. Most diets are a sprint, but weight loss that lasts is a marathon. Lifestyle changes last the rest of your life. A quick-fix diet lasts only as long as it gives you results (or you give up on it, whichever comes first) but it won't pull you through the stretch. Gimmicky diets—as opposed to just eating moderately and healthfully—are not sustainable.

So, I recommend making small changes, one, maybe two at a time. Make one change a week, and by the end of the year, you've made 52. Now that's significant! Instead of overhauling your whole diet in one week, for instance, just start with breakfast. If you always order a tall mocha drink and big blueberry muffin, or even something seemingly healthy (but fattening) like a big bowl of granola, change it up. Forget the mocha and just get a regular cup of coffee. To eat, try an all-fruit smoothie (no added sherbet like they put in at most smoothie stores) or a bowl of steel-cut oatmeal (without the brown sugar and cream). Just fix breakfast, nothing else. Try that for a week, then move on to lunch. Inch by inch, you'll eventually make over your whole diet.

||||||||||||||||||||||||||||||||||||||||||||||||||||||||||||||||||||||||

Small Victories Add Up

So I've been feeling pretty frustrated because my scale has been stubborn for three weeks straight. . . . I kinda wanna throw it out the window. But today, I had two great nonscale victories: First, several people from work independently asked me what I'm doing because I'm looking "skinny" and "lean." And second, I had to run down the hall and up three flights of stairs and I was fine—not even a little winded after. Amazing!

—Delia, posted on *The Revolution* Facebook page

Now, it is true that some people can handle making bigger, cold-turkey-types of changes and manage to stick to them. I love the approach that *The Biggest Loser* contestant named Tony took. One of the first changes he made—and he made it before he even got on the show—was to give up fast food. And believe me, this was significant. "I had a whole wallet dedicated to fast food," says Tony. "I had a buy-one-get-one-free coupon for every fast-food restaurant there is. And I'd eat both of the meals." In fact, fast food was his life. His first job ever was at a fast-food restaurant, and over several decades, he worked up to manager, so his meals were always free.

In Tony's case, taking that one big step led to another. Next, he decided to exercise, but gyms were expensive and, he was so big that they were dismissive of him when he expressed a desire to work out. So he walked. "Two hours in the morning and 2 hours every evening. By the time I got on the show, I'd already lost 30 pounds." Four hours a day wasn't a small change, but the point is that even though Tony's changes weren't small, they were incremental. He didn't take it all on at once. (By the way, the fact that Tony made changes before the show started was unusual. Most contestants would eat like crazy before the show started to pump up the pounds and make their weight loss seem even more dramatic.)

What small and/or incremental changes give you are small victories, and I advise savoring every one. It can be something tiny ("I walked into my colleague's office and didn't grab anything out of her candy bowl") or bigger ("I increased the resistance on the weight machines"). It doesn't matter. Make a note of every single one. We ask cast members to write down their small victories each day, and one of the best ones I ever heard was this: "I tried today even when my trainer wasn't looking." Most people would gloss over that victory, but when I heard that, I read it to the whole group. "Here's what this guy is really saying," I told them. "When no one was looking before, he wasn't his best as a father, his best as a worker, his best as a husband, his best as a human being. Think about that. That's what he just said. But today, he said that even when no one was looking, he gave his best. Is he now going to try harder as a father, a worker, a husband, a human being? If he does, it will be a much greater victory than whatever his numbers on the scale end up being. That is real transformation."

The little victories that come from making small changes can alter your life in so many big ways. They show you that you can do things you never thought you could do, and that, in turn, helps give you the confidence you need to improve the overall quality of your life. Suddenly, you're not just increasing the resistance on the weights, you're decreasing the amount of time it takes you to do your work; now you have more time to spend with your friends or your kids. Now you're not just turning down a colleague's candy, you're turning down a colleague's efforts to foist his work on you. Little acts of willpower and accomplishment generate confidence. I can't tell you how many of our cast members leave the show dreaming big. For instance, Robert and Raymond, the twins who supported their whole family while their mother was in jail, began thinking about leaving their jobs at the door and window factory and embarking on new careers—in the health and fitness field. "Learning the things that I could do changed how I looked at myself 100 percent," says Robert.

The thing about small victories is that they have a very positive cumulative effect. Panda, who was so successful at weight loss he hit his goal before leaving Boot Camp, describes what the progression was like for him. "After one day, you say to yourself, 'I'm strong enough to be able to do this for a day.' That one day becomes two days, which becomes a week, which becomes two weeks, which becomes a month." Everything for him was, sometimes literally, putting one foot in front of the other.

We take all the *Extreme Weight Loss* Boot Camp participants to Red Rocks, an amphitheater near Denver, where we have them work out on the stairs. The first time out, standing at the bottom, looking up at the top, Panda panicked and said to himself, "There is no way I can climb all the way up without stopping." But then he thought, *but I can take one step. And that one step will lead me to the next.* Looking back, he says, "sometimes, you're so focused on what's off in the distance and that big number when what you really need to do is focus on what you're doing right now. It's like that Chinese proverb: A journey of a hundred miles begins with a single step."

Ultimately, that means stay present in the moment. Don't let the future overwhelm you. Live in the moment, and appreciate every goal you hit and every victory you achieve. You might not realize it, but you are slowly retraining your brain to release that feel-good chemical dopamine not just when you eat chocolate cake, but when you make healthy, positive steps in your life. So be focused, be purposeful. Think about today, not tomorrow.

CHAPTER 14

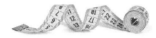

Shake Up Your Life

A lot of people—especially people who have tried out for our shows—are walking around in a coma. They're the walking dead. They just keep going through the motions, doing the same things day after day. They're so used to their routines, their habits—what has become of their lives—that they don't see the truth. Until someone says, "Hey, look around," they don't even know that something is wrong. In fact, many cast members are shocked at how much they weigh when they have their first weigh-in. They know they're overweight, but not how serious it has become. When you gain a pound a week, you just don't notice. But then 100 weeks go by, and you're 100 pounds heavier. When someone points it out, you're blindsided. You haven't even noticed. Like I said, the walking dead.

Habit is an enemy for skinny people, too. I mean bad habits, of course, but also just plain old habit. You buy the same things at the grocery store. You come home after work and do the same thing night after night. You go to the same restaurants. You do the same activities with your family or friends on the weekend. Most times, you don't even realize that you're stuck in a rut. It's *Groundhog Day* all over again. If you have a great Groundhog Day, who wouldn't want to repeat it? But if you don't have a good Groundhog Day and things in your life aren't going well, it's hell. Another day, and I'm still not happy with my husband, my kids are still not nice to me, my bank account is still teetering on the edge—you have to numb yourself and go through the motions. So, it's no wonder that people slowly get into a routine and turn their brains off. But, little by little, that routine can get you in trouble.

Just to drive home the point that a lot of people are on autopilot, let me tell you this story from one of our shows. We had two people, a couple about to be married, that we had decided to cast on the show, but they didn't know it yet. Our idea was to surprise them at their favorite restaurant on Bourbon Street in New Orleans, so we hid cameras all around the place in order to catch what we expected to be their last extravagantly decadent meal. As the cameras rolled, the two of them ordered all their usual greasy, fattening dishes—triple sliders and a side of fries with all the extras (sour cream, guacamole, and more) on top. The portions, by the way, were huge. But instead of just playing it straight, we decided to play a little trick on them by sabotaging the food they'd ordered. Then Heidi and Chris would pop out and say, "Surprise! You're on the show, and you're never going to eat this stuff again." We thought it would be funny; we didn't expect the result we got.

Heidi and Chris went into the kitchen and poured mounds of salt, hot sauce, and Cajun seasonings on the food, doing their best to make the food inedible. It was gross. We thought the couple would take one bite, be repulsed, and welcome the idea that they'd never eat that stuff again. As we watched, they ate the first bites of fries. No reaction. Then the sliders. Again, no reaction. Pretty soon, they were digging into the entire meal, moaning with sounds of joy. It was then that we realized that they didn't even taste it! All that indulging wasn't about the food. It was the habit, the ritual; maybe the memory of what that food tasted like at some pivotal point in their lives. Because it sure wasn't about the food, which would have caused most people to gag. That's sleepwalking through life.

It's taken for granted that to lose weight, you need to change your eating and exercise habits. Of course, you have to stop doing things like going to get a triple mocha latte two or three times a day. But I say do more. Change up some of the things that seem to have nothing to do with weight loss, and you will drop pounds. Because what you're trying to do here is make a better life for yourself; eating and exercise is just one part of that. It's like dominos; changing one thing will help you change the next and the next and the next. Pretty soon you're living a different life. Here's another metaphor for you: If you do the same biceps exercise every single time you go to the gym, your biceps muscles will adapt and stop getting stronger. They're used to the same thing. To get those muscles to grow, you have to shock them by doing something different. Maybe, for instance, instead of doing curls each workout session, you spend some time on the rowing machine to work your arms in a different way. Same thing if you're a runner. You run the same direction and speed every time, you'll never get any faster or improve your stamina. Start doing sprint intervals, or make each day you run a different intensity and distance, and, suddenly, you get better and faster. Life works the same way.

Okay, so here's what I want you to do to shake up your life. Go into your bedroom and take everything out. I'm not talking about just cleaning it up. Empty the room completely; deep clean it. Then sit in the empty room in silence. Look around you. A clean slate. A new beginning. What do you feel? Does the room feel bigger? Does it feel like a new space? Live with it like this for a few hours. Start thinking creatively. Should the bed go on the opposite wall? Do you really need that 20-year-old table you have been using just to pile up unopened mail? Should the room be a different color? Breathe deep in the calm of it all. Now go outside the room, look at what you've removed, and judge it all. Put it in three piles: must have, get rid of, and not sure. Immediately throw out everything that fell into the get-rid-of pile. Now go back and separate the rest into three piles again; hopefully you'll find even more to give away.

After you have done this, put your room back together, changing everything. Put the bed on a different wall. Move the artwork. Maybe get rid of a few things and, if you're up for it, buy some new things. It probably sounds crazy or maybe even a waste of time. When I suggest it to people, they're usually skeptical. "I want to lose weight, so I go into my bedroom and empty everything out? No, no, I said I want to lose weight." Right. I got it, but this is part of it. Most people will tell you that to get a fresh start, you should go take everything out of your kitchen cupboards and refrigerator, and yes, of course, that can help. But leave that for a while. First get to the bedroom (or living room; that works, too). Taking everything out and doing a deep clean is essentially what I'm asking you to do to yourself, too. Take a look around. That is called waking yourself up, and that requires more than just eating better. Doing a deep clean of your home is the first step to doing a deep clean of your mind.

I can't claim to really know the science behind this, but I know that I've seen what happens when people shake things up. It's like they're rewiring they're brains—changing the pathways—and it helps them break habits and feel differently not just about their space, but about themselves. When you make over your living space, instead of walking back in and automatically going back to your old ways, this visual and spatial disruption will make life seem different—and it will be different now. You're different now—different eating habits, different activity habits, a different way of thinking.

One of the most depressing moments for me as a producer was when we sent a cast member named Rodney home after his 90-day weigh-in. There was a giant celebration. Hundreds of people had come out to scream his name, applaud him, and high-five him.

Then, on a high from all the love surrounding him, he walked up to his apartment door, opened it, and the camera followed him into the place that looked exactly as he'd left it 90 days earlier. He walked right into all the old feelings of failure as embodied by that crappy apartment. Our brains make associations. We're like Pavlov's dogs, so when we walk into a room, our subconscious links it to expectations. And it's pretty powerful. So if you've always sat around in your living room kicking back in the recliner downing caramel corn after a brutal day at work, or crawled into bed with a carton of cookie-dough ice cream because you didn't want to face your family, those urges are going to resurface every time you set eyes on that same old space.

|||||||||||||||||||||||||||||||||||||||||||||||||||||||||||||||||||||||||||

Change Is Motivating

Hi, JD,

One of the best pieces of advice that you've given that sticks in my head is to change your living environment. With each phase I have changed my home, recreating spaces from home gyms to a home office to a sewing room. After the finale, I came back and changed my space again and when I came home from surgery I did it once more. Each time I feel complacent I change my environment and it keeps me motivated. Thank you for that tip.

My life has completely changed and I am appreciative that you have selected me to go through this transformation so that I could live the life I've always wanted to live.

—Kim, *Extreme Weight Loss* cast member, via email

I know this sounds like mumbo jumbo, but it's not. I've seen it so many times. Redecorating a room is like redecorating your mind, and it makes a significant difference. That's what Rodney did. He changed his bedroom around; soon after, he fell in love. And he kept off almost all the weight he lost on the show. You can go even further with this. Change the way you drive to work. Change where you go on your lunch hour. Choose different activities on the weekend. If you walk around the block clockwise, do it counterclockwise. If you usually eat on the couch, eat at the table instead. If you eat at the table, change the seat you usually sit at. Make your life as different as possible, and it will be easier to break the habit of picking up a daily double mochaccino with extra whip or always ordering the cheesecake for dessert. Think of it as retraining your brain. You don't have to make a zillion changes at once; in fact, I would make them one at a time (remember: dream big, but act small). You don't want to overwhelm yourself. If you can't keep up with a bunch of changes, you're just going to feel bad about yourself, and you know where that leads . . . to the nearest fast food drive-thru.

And don't discount the power of one change; it can have an unexpected impact. I'll give you an example, not weight-related, but habit-related nonetheless. When one of my sons was younger, he came into our bedroom every night. From the time he could walk until he was nine years old, he'd appear nightly and get into our bed. No joke, 7 days a week for 9 years. We tried everything to get him to stop. Finally, we put a little mattress at the end of our bed so he'd get the message that he couldn't sleep *in* our bed. It went on so long that I figured that by the time he was in high school, he'd be bringing his girlfriend with him. It was that bad. But surprisingly when he was nine, we moved to a new house, and he just never did it again. We never talked about it. We never said, "In the new house, you can't do that anymore." The change just snapped his behavior naturally.

Shake-ups have unexpected consequences and, certainly in the case of weight loss, that's a good thing. I particularly believe that making changes that lead to a better-organized life can make it easier to get the pounds off. I may be a little OCD myself, but I've seen it enough times to confidently say that disorder in one area of life makes it difficult to attain order in another area of life.

A few years ago, we had the financial guru Suze Orman on *The Biggest Loser*. We often brought experts in various areas onto the show, and Suze was one of them. Before she met with the contestants, she asked us to get everyone's credit score.

"Why?" I asked her. "Why would you need their credit scores?"

She said, "I'm convinced that I can pick the winner of the show based on their credit scores."

"How is that even possible?" I replied.

"If you can't count your money, you probably can't count calories either," said Suze.

I was skeptical, but we got her everyone's credit score anyway. We had actually planned for her to do something completely different on the show, but once she asked for the FICO scores, we changed her segment to deal with credit. She called out the people with low scores, admonishing them, then turned to the person with the highest score and predicted a win. It was only week two of the competition, but she was convinced that she already knew who the winner was. In the end, six months later, she ended up being right! She pegged it in week two of a six-month competition!

And I came to see what she was talking about. If you're sinking under the craziness of your life, not paying bills, letting debt pile up, it's not surprising that you're also sinking under the weight of your body. Suze believed that the person with the highest FICO score would also be the person most capable of staying on the plan. A person capable of balancing her checkbook, she reasoned, was also going to be able to handle the math involved with calorie counting and interval training. Someone who could focus on financial stability could also focus on the road to recovery.

In what other areas of your life are you asleep at the wheel? Look at everything. How do you rank as a parent, a worker, a spouse? Do you let your mail pile up so high that it's a chore to open it? Do you procrastinate when it comes to fixing things around your house? These are all signs of a sleepy brain. Wake it up—and infuse it with a new sense of purpose and passion! Be willing to make changes, take action, and nothing will stand in your way.

||||||||||||||||||||||||||||||||||||||||||||||||||||||||||||||||||||||||||||||

Change Is Good!

Hi JD,

I was reflecting upon the past year, and I still can't believe how I could not see how truly "broken" I was. If it wasn't for the show, I don't think I would have ever emerged from my patterns of self-destruction.

The physical weight loss is such a gift but is trumped by the mental and spiritual clarity I gained.

Self-hatred and unforgiveness are extremely powerful emotions that consumed me for years, and stole my joy. This process has restored my joy, and I cannot be any happier to rediscover the old Jackie.

Everyone I run into tells me there is an energy and light when I enter the room. This makes me so happy that others can see what I genuinely feel.

I remember you told us all to go home and makes changes. I wholeheartedly took your advice. I made a new space in my home office dedicated to display my running bibs from all the competitions I have completed. I call it my wall of motivation.

I also recently made a huge change with my career. I resigned my good-paying job with the D.A.'s office to pursue a job in the health and wellness field. Beginning August, I will be working for Lifetime Fitness. I want to motivate people to become fit and healthy, and let them know anything is possible.

—Jackie, *Extreme Weight Loss* cast member, via email

CHAPTER 15

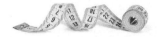

Get an Education in Nutrition

We get two types of people on our shows: People who know *everything* about food, and people who know *nothing* about food. Yet even the know-it-alls can always use a course in nutrition. Their brains are like a calorie database—they can tell you the number of calories in a single lettuce leaf (virtually none)—and they may even know a little about fats and carbs, but they still really don't know how to eat healthfully (it's what you put on the lettuce leaf that's the problem). These are the people that think eating diet TV dinners every night is a good choice. Calorie-wise, maybe, but do you know how many chemicals and grams of sodium are in those highly processed packaged foods? If you don't, you need to find out. Put simply, processed anything is not the best choice for your health.

Have you noticed that obesity rates leap up with a vengeance every time a new food trend is shoved into our consciousness? The food revolution was supposed to make our lives better, but it actually has made it worse. First, in the 1950s, it was convenience foods like TV dinners (better for the start of the age of working mothers), then came the proliferation of fast-food places in the 1970s—it wasn't just McDonald's anymore but Taco Bell, KFC, Popeye's, Chik-fil-A, and Arby's, all of them eventually supersizing their meals and sodas (and helping the family on the go who needed to eat quickly). Next, in the 1980s, the notion that we should eat fat-free foods took hold. What did they do to make our foods fat-free? Added sugar! And lots of it! Carbs were in; carbs were out. It's like a virus, growing in power and infecting more and more people with each new invention. First the government says eat lots of meat. Now, research is saying meat is a carcinogen and we're eating way too much sugar. Eat a plant-based diet, they (finally!) say. It's not only better for you but it will help us sustain the Earth.

|||||||||||||||||||||||||||||||||||||||||||||||||||||||||||||||||||||||||||||||||||||||

When You become a Person Who Eats Healthfully, Everything Changes

Confession: I cheated today! I had my vinaigrette dressing tossed into my salad instead of dipping it on the side. Isn't it crazy that our perception of "cheating" has changed? LOL.

—Jamilla, posted on *The Revolution* Facebook page

My point is that it's very confusing. And even when solid nutrition information is laid out straight, there are areas of the country where the message is still not getting through. Classic example: Before Bruce came on the show, he owned a monster 100-ounce mug that he would fill with soda at least three times a day. That's the equivalent of more than four of those big 2-liter bottles. How many calories do you think that is? A 2-liter bottle of soda has about 800 to 900 calories. Multiply that by the number of times Bruce was refilling the container and he's drinking in between 3,000 and 4,000 calories a day, more than the amount most people *eat*—and at least one and a half times more than his current calorie intake for the day. He was horrified when he found out. Soda is one of our worst enemies—regular or diet—it makes no difference (yes, there's a calorie difference but diet soda just makes you crave more sweet stuff). If you haven't already, give up soda now.

In my book you should *never* drink a calorie other than the occasional alcoholic drink (and you shouldn't even do that if you're trying to lose weight). News flash. Drink water. The planet and humans are mostly made of it. It makes sense to drink something that we are made of. I know what you are saying to yourself. But I love the feel of the fizz on the back on my throat. Yeah, yeah, and the scientists that work for the big soft drink companies designed it that way. You drink it, and they win. Sodas are completely empty calories. I would rather see you eat a cookie than drink a soda. That's how much I dislike soda! If you love fizz so much, have a club soda.

Like Bruce, Robert and Raymond also had no sense of how many calories they were taking in. By their own account, they'd eat fast food four, five, even six times a day. They knew it wasn't great, but they'd tell themselves, "It's meat and a tortilla; it's not horrible for you." During their time on *Extreme Weight Loss*, Robert started doing a little investigating, and was shocked to find that the burritos he was eating totaled about 3,000 calories, not counting the extras on the side. To my mind, as horrifying as all those calories are, the ingredients (truckloads of sodium and unhealthy fats) are worse.

Some mistakes people make are less blatant. "I mostly eat salads," a cast member will tell me, beaming about her good choice. The fact that her salads are usually drenched in thick white dressing, sprinkled with cheese, and littered with croutons doesn't seem to register. If soda is the recognizable scourge of America, salad is the sneaky enemy that masquerades as a friend—and ranch dressing is its accomplice. Even olive oil, which is known as a "healthy fat," can be a problem. One tablespoon of olive oil is 120 calories of pure fat. How many people do you know who put only one tablespoon of olive oil on an entire salad? So watch out for salads that have anything more than a good assortment of lettuce and other vegetables and a light coating of dressing. Keep it colorful: Anything white in a salad (i.e., blue cheese dressing, ranch, cheese) other than cauliflower is adding calories you don't need.

At first, your taste buds will scream for that ranch dressing. Don't give in to them. Within days, your taste buds will stop longing for that ranch. Believe it or not, a salad with fresh lemon juice or balsamic vinegar and a touch of oil will be more enticing to you than ever before.

Salads and soda. That's about as specific as I'm going to get here; as you know, this isn't a diet book. This is a book about using your brain to lose weight. But I do want to talk about how important it is to get your overall nutrition facts straight. Your action steps in regard to eating shouldn't just focus on what you should take out of your diet; it should also concentrate on what you should add in. Learn about both. Taking unhealthy calories out, putting healthy calories in.

|||||||||||||||||||||||||||||||||||||||||||||||||||||||||||||||||||||||||

What Tastes Better Than Chocolate Cake? Resisting Chocolate Cake

Reporting live from the West Coast,

Yesterday was major! My absolute favorite cake in the world is chocolate cake with white frosting! We had a project team celebration, and what do you think they served. . . . chocolate cake with white frosting! I am so very proud to report, *I did not have any! Not even a crumb!* I ate a Healthy Choice fudge bar—100 calories and 5 grams of sugar! Thanks for keeping me accountable and inspired!

—Stacey, posted on *The Revolution* Facebook page

These days, it's pretty easy to find out how many calories are in just about any food you're eating. Many casual restaurants provide nutrition information (as do fast-food restaurants—if you want to see how out of control your calories are, just go to your favorite fast-food restaurant's website) and, of course, all food packages must be labeled. But here's the thing. It's so easy to misconstrue label information. A package of crackers may say you'll be taking in 100 calories—if you nibble at *one-fifth* of the package, but who notices the serving size? And who eats one-fifth of the package? Before you know it, you've wolfed down 500 calories.

Some foods *seem* healthy, but that doesn't mean they're not fattening. A quick look at the label of one brand of kale chips shows it has 640 calories. Kale! So be careful.

When there's no nutrition information available, you can find yourself entering a danger zone. Even our nutrition team was shocked when we had the well-known chef Rocco DiSpirito on an episode of *Extreme Weight Loss,* and he gave us a peek into what goes on behind the scenes in a restaurant kitchen.

Every night, his restaurant would serve 100 people. "I'd start the night with 16 pounds of butter at my station," said Rocco. That sounded like a lot, but maybe not terrible if you divided it by 100 people. Then Rocco landed the knockout punch. "And there were *four* of me!"

Can you imagine how much butter that is? Do the math: 64 pounds of butter divided by 100 people = 0.64 pound or about 2,000 calories per person—and that's not including the food that came along with all that butter! As they cooked, the chefs would grab and grab and grab at those hunks of butter, putting it in everything. By the night's end, every ounce of the butter was gone—and the customers were happy. Who wouldn't be? Butter makes everything taste delicious, and they'd just eaten a great meal without the guilt of knowing that they'd just devoured more than a half-pound of butter each. Put enough butter on the book you are reading now, and I bet that would taste good, too!

I'll let you in on another secret we learned: About half the time you ask your restaurant server to hold the butter or oil, the kitchen ignores your request. If your meal tastes suspiciously succulent despite your pleas for no oil or butter, you are probably being duped. Chefs are more concerned about their food tasting good and developing a customer following than they are about your health. It's a business!

I once heard a cautionary tale about a very famous woman who was a regular at a swanky Hollywood watering hole run by a chef who was just as famous as she was. The woman was trying to watch her weight and asked the chef to make her pasta without butter or oil. He goes back into the kitchen and, a short while later, presents her with a fantastic dish that she says is the greatest pasta she's ever had. She loves it so much that she orders it again the following week. This time, though, the famous chef isn't there so the chef on duty makes the no-butter, no-oil pasta she asks for. This time, though, it tastes terrible. She sends it back and demands that they make it the way the famous chef had. Frantic, they call him on the phone. "How did you make that no-butter, no-oil pasta?" The famous chef starts laughing. "I made it the exact same way I always make it. I just told her it didn't have butter or oil!" Let that be a warning to you!

As long as you don't go out to restaurants and order pasta every night, eating nutritiously can be very simple. Here's a rule of thumb: Eat only what is grown or raised in or on the Earth and presented to you without processing. That means unadulterated fruits, vegetables, and, rarely if ever, sustainably (and conscientiously) produced eggs, poultry, seafood, and meat. Just limiting the amount of packages you open alone will make a difference in how much you weigh and how you feel. (Try the exercises on page 225 and page 241, and you'll see what I mean.)

And there's some evidence that more and more people are clueing in to this fact. Recently the *New York Times* reported that sales of soda and sugary cereals are down as is the revenue of some fast food operations. Many big food companies are dropping artificial flavors and preservatives and, by buying up smaller companies that produce healthy, organic edibles, casting their lot in the direction of healthier products. Even sales of fruits and vegetables are up!

To me, the most important part of the transformation process is not the actual pounds you lose, but the renovation of your health, mentally and physically. So while calories have to be considered, of course, think about all the benefits good food can give you, and stop eating crap. To look at the participants in our shows, you'd never think they were malnourished, but amazingly, most of them are. They're eating so poorly, living on cheese sticks, processed chicken fingers, soda, and corn chips, that some of them are even anemic. They eat thousands of calories but get zero nutrition. By nutrition, I mean vitamins and minerals, fiber, and all the micronutrients that experts tell us help prevent disease. That's what you get when you eat whole, unprocessed foods. Fresh, nutritionally dense foods that come from the Earth (not a lab!) are all that should go in your mouth. If you can't always get fresh, frozen fruits and veggies are better than canned. They are picked at the peak of ripeness and frozen right away so they retain more of their nutrients.

There are so many benefits from eating mostly plant foods. Have you heard of the China Study? In 2005, the world-renowned Cornell University researcher T. Colin Campbell published the results of a 20-year joint investigation by Cornell, Oxford University, and the Chinese Academy of Preventive Medicine that found eating animal-based foods is associated with chronic disease. The study also found that people who ate primarily plant-based diets were far healthier—they had virtually no incidence of heart disease, stroke, or diabetes and very low rates of cancer. Campbell and his colleagues have even found that you can reverse disease by switching to a plant-based diet. So why aren't we all doing it?

When you make the transition, you are also going to naturally lose weight. In one of his many studies, Campbell also looked at the effects of a diet low in saturated fat and refined carbohydrates and high in fresh fruits, vegetables, beans, and nuts. The results were impressive: The people who changed over to the plant-based, nutritionally dense diet lost an average of 31 pounds. When they came back two years later, they'd lost an average of 53 pounds. Wow!

My own family has switched to a mostly plant-based diet. Even the U.S. government, the most conservative body there is, is now advocating that people eat far less meat and are working on changing the food guidelines. Meat is bad for our health, it's bad for the environment, and it's not sustainable. Sugar, refined carbs, and fat are generally the problem for people who need to lose weight, but if you're a big meat-eater, ratchet it back. A life existing on hamburgers is good for no one. Even cutting your meat portion in half and increasing the amount of veggies on the plate is a huge step in the right direction.

At the same time, I urge you not to get carried away with calorie reduction. I've seen people go overboard, to their detriment. One of our cast members started to lose weight really rapidly, actually at an alarming rate. It turned out that he had stopped eating regular meals and was living on protein bars and a handful of almonds here and there. That was the worst idea ever. He was nervous that his lack of nutrition knowledge was going to hurt him, so he just went with a food that was approved of by the show's dietitian: protein bars. Approved of, yes, but for emergency situations, not as a main source of calories. When it's not getting enough nourishment, your body will cannibalize its own muscle tissue. We put the guy in the Bod Pod, a machine that measures body composition, and discovered that he had lost 10 to 15 pounds of muscle. I want you to lose fat, not muscle! This process is about getting healthy. Don't just think that dropping weight will make you healthy. It takes a lot more.

Know yourself, not just nutrition. Knowing your nutrition facts is going to help you make better choices, but you still have to deal with issues of control. Can you resist favorite foods put right in front of you? Then do your best to make sure they *aren't* right in front of you. I would argue that sometimes you don't actually need willpower if you consistently make the right choice. If there's nothing "dangerous" in your house, you don't have to worry about making a bad choice. If you have to get in your car when it's 18 degrees Fahrenheit outside to get a carton of ice cream, you're not going to get it (at least most of you won't). But if you're snuggled up in your warm house next to the fire, settled in to binge watch a show on Netflix, and there's a half-gallon in your house, you're eating the whole thing. A skinny person would, too. And if you do get in your car to brave the 18-degree weather, talk to yourself all the way there and decide BEFORE you get there what you are ordering. Then keep your promise. If you go in with an open mind, you will end up in the ice cream shop with an open mouth. My trick is to tell my wife in the car that I'm getting the kid's scoop so I don't turn into a hypocrite once I get into the ice cream shop. That is being in control of your destiny!

Until you form new habits, take temptation out of the equation. If you need to put a padlock on your refrigerator and give the key to your husband or neighbor so you won't eat at night, do it. I am not kidding here. Remove temptation, because you are human. Would you put a bottle of gin next to an alcoholic and ask him to only have one shot a day? So why would you put a half-gallon of ice cream in front of a food addict and ask her to only have one spoonful a day?

Can't resist eating everything on your plate? Open up the salt-shaker and pour salt all over your food after you've eaten half. Don't just throw the remaining Thin Mint Girl Scout cookies in the trash after you've eaten two or three, destroy them with hot water—because you know you're going to dig them out of the garbage if you don't. These things sound crazy (and wasteful), and maybe they are, but what you're doing is training yourself to eat better so that, eventually, as you develop new, healthier habits, exercising restraint isn't going to be such a big deal for you. Set yourself up for success, and you'll win.

Another way to set yourself up for success is to always plan ahead. Even if you're going to be eating out, check out the restaurant menu on Yelp or on the restaurant's website first. Decide what you're going to have before you go, and you'll be less likely to order something you shouldn't. If one reason you end up in the drive-thru line at McDonald's is because you're pressed for time during the week, plan your meals and make food on the weekend. Bring your lunch to work. These are the basics of being a healthy eater, while being caught unprepared is what leads people to make bad choices 90 percent of the time. I've seen this play out on our shows, but I'm not the only one who's noticed. When Oprah's *O* magazine analyzed data from MyFitnessPal, the online weight-loss tool, they found that the users who'd lost 30 pounds or more were twice as likely to plan their meals and snacks ahead of time as people who'd only lost a little weight.

Twice as likely! Don't reinvent the wheel here. Do what other successful people do. Follow patterns that work, and shockingly you will find they work for you, too. I asked one of our very successful weight-loss contestants what he tells people when they ask his secret for losing weight. You know what he said? "Turns out eating better and moving more really works." He lost more than 200 pounds by doing the basics.

Of course, there will be times when you won't be able to plan ahead or control your environment. Life happens. That's where you need to work that willpower you've been developing—and see if you can be happy with less. My favorite ice cream shop has a great thing called the itsy bitsy. It's just about a large spoonful of ice cream in a tiny cone. Sometimes after dinner, we'll walk over and get an itsy bitsy, and it's great. We feel like we've had the whole ice cream shop experience—standing in line with the crowd, watching our kids flip-flop back and forth about what flavor they're going to get—but we go home no worse for it. I have my itsy bitsy, and it's enough. It's plenty. We had the experience, and that's what we're after. And it cost us only about 100 calories to do it. So if it is the experience and the act of going to the ice cream store and smelling the fresh-made cones, and seeing the excited kids in the line, then go do it. But *commit* ahead of time to what you are going to get (write it down if you have to) and under no circumstances deviate from your plan.

One of the things that makes the experience satisfying is that the itsy bitsy is the real thing. I'm not a big believer in most low-calorie, "diet" versions of food. Usually, these are foods that have chemical flavor enhancers or are bolstered with sugar. Many of them are also lightened up in such a way that they aren't satisfying. If you want pizza, get a slice of pizza (just don't eat the whole pie). Eating pizza with light cheese is just going to make you crave more pizza. You may even end up eating the real thing on top of the diet slice you just ate. It's the same thing with diet soda. Why do I hate it so much? It doesn't have calories. But it does have chemicals and an intensely sweet taste that just makes you long for more. You may never wean yourself off sweets if you drink diet soda.

Here's something to think about, too. Don't let money drive your eating decisions. (Ironically, it used to be that being fat was a sign of wealth. Back when kings had big bellies, it was because they were at the top of the food chain, feasting on whatever they wanted, while the poor peasants went hungry.) When I get the itsy bitsy at my neighborhood ice cream shop, I never feel like I got gypped. Yeah, it probably cost me more than sticking a spoon into a carton in my freezer, but it's worth it not to have the temptation at home.

In one of our *Extreme Weight Loss* episodes, we filmed another couple in a restaurant with a hidden camera right before they were going to get surprised by Chris and Heidi, who'd be telling them they'd been picked for the show. The guy was sitting at the table with 30 saucy, greasy chicken wings in front of him. His fiancée says to him (and the guy, by the way, was 450 pounds), "Don't eat those. We really need to start our diets now."

"Yeah, you're right," he replied, "But I paid for these!" That was his mentality. *I paid for these, so I have to eat them.* That is just so wrong. Losing the price of a batch of chicken wings is so insignificant compared to what you lose when you completely disrespect your body. And besides, once you stop eating so much, you're going to save money in the long run. Think about the future, not the here and now.

I fall into the camp that thinks you should settle into a way of eating and stick with it. Deviating a little here and there might be okay, but if your personal rules are that you don't eat fattening, processed, unhealthy food then you don't eat fattening . . . you get my drift. Changing your eating habits is like giving up drugs and alcohol. In 12-step lingo, it's called "working the program," and you have to do it every day.

Something we have cast members do that I think is extremely beneficial is to keep a food log. Moses probably kept a food log—that's how long this recommendation has been around—but there's good reason for it. You don't really know the cold hard facts of how much you're eating until you see it in black-and-white. Whether you do it on your computer with the help of an online weight-loss tool or whether you just get a notebook and start recording every morsel that passes your lips, it's going to help hold you accountable—even if you're just reporting it to yourself. (And you don't have to just report it to yourself; go ahead and post your daily entries on Facebook where other people can see them. Now that will really hold you accountable). Everything—every piece of gum, every bite you take from someone else's plate, every piece of candy you find in the recesses of your desk drawer, everything—goes into that log. Sometimes, you will choose not to eat that extra snack, because you are too lazy to go over and enter it in your log.

So start writing. *And be honest!* If you're not going to be honest with yourself, there's no point in doing it. So while facing up to what you're really eating can be scary, you can't change things about yourself if you don't have all the facts. Get the facts, then deal with them.

CHAPTER 16

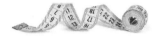

Learn to Love Exercise

If you think you can never love working out, let me tell you more of Amber's story. Amber, whom you'll remember was on *Extreme Weight Loss* with her fiancé, absolutely hated exercise. Asked to describe herself, she'd say she was an indoor girl. "I love to read. I love movies. I love snuggling with my dog on the couch. I have never been one to say, 'Let's go for a hike,'" she told me. Part of this might have been rebellion. Amber grew up in a family that was health conscious and active. Her stepfather was especially diligent. "He's Mr. Fitness, in his sixties and still does short board surfing daily," she says, "My mom and I laugh at him because he eats chicken and broccoli for lunch every single day."

Amber was definitely the slacker in the family so, for her, the first weeks of Boot Camp were pretty torturous. The expectation that she work out for hours every day made her grouchy and argumentative. She'd pick fights with her fiancé, Bryce, who took to the exercise part much more easily. It wasn't as though Amber had never exercised before, at least in theory. In high school, she'd joined the swim team because it didn't involve running, which she hated even more than swimming. Plus, with swimming, she figured she could train inconspicuously in the slow lane and that nobody would pay her much mind; they'd see she had no potential—if they saw her at all. Because more often than not, after Amber's mom drove her to the 5:00 a.m. practice, Amber would slip into the locker room and stay there. "I was the queen of ditching practice," she says.

On *Extreme Weight Loss*, Amber couldn't ditch her workouts without some serious flack. So she did them, unhappily at first. One way she got through them was to remind herself that every workout has an end. It became her mantra. Ten more minutes left to go on the treadmill? *Every workout has an end.* Five more sit-ups? *Every workout has an end.* "Then when it was done, I would think, 'That wasn't so bad,'" she says. "It was like I had amnesia."

Then something weird happened (weird to Amber's mind, not to mine because I've seen it a thousand times). Typically, when anything sent Amber into an emotional tailspin, she'd drown herself in food. When she was 13, her 40-year-old father became engaged to a woman who was 21, closer in age to Amber than to her father. It upset her, but she didn't feel comfortable voicing her opinion. Along with internalizing her feelings, she "internalized" about 30 chocolate bars she was supposed to be selling to raise money for school. Amber hid in the closet, devoured the chocolate, then stuffed the wrappers in her dresser. When her mother found them while putting away the laundry, she sobbed. As someone who once only found solace in food, Amber was stunned to discover that, upset one day during Boot Camp, she wanted to run, not eat. She ran and ran until that bubbling feeling of distress subsided. She looked at her watch. She'd run for an *hour*. Suddenly, Amber understood what all those runners were talking about. She understood runner's high. "It kind of caught me off-guard. Ever since then, it's been my go-to for anxiety," says Amber.

This can happen to you. It might not be running for an hour without stopping, it might not be running at all, but you will find the turning point. One reason I believe that Amber did is because she kept at exercise long enough to reap its rewards. Exercise never feels good in the beginning, even for me, and I run several times a week. But if you give up after 15 minutes and say, "This isn't for me," you're never going to experience all that exercise can do for you. You'll never get that endorphin rush. You'll never see your body start to change. You'll never show yourself that you can master a challenge. But tough it out like Amber did, and you will be as pleasantly surprised as she was. "I always thought you were born liking exercise," says Amber, "that you had a special thing inside you. When I'd hear people on other *Extreme Weight Loss* episodes say, 'I love working out,' I'd think, okay, you're clearly crazy. But I think it's just letting it sneak up on you."

You (Yes, You), Too, Can Learn to Love Exercise

Hey everyone,

I just faced my fear in spin class! I woke up at 4:30 a.m. and said today is the day . . . I took my first-ever spin class. It started at 5:15 a.m., and I burned 807 calories! OMG . . . I loved it. It was fun and challenging all at the same time. I am actually in shape. I did it; I did it! I am so proud of me today!

—Angela, posted on *The Revolution* Facebook page

The other thing that Amber did to her everlasting benefit was to try a lot of different types of exercise. There are so many forms of physical activity. *Something* is going to click if you just give it a chance. For Amber, it was hit and miss, and that's to be expected. She played ultimate football (fun, but she wasn't going to make it a regular thing), Zumba (she learned she had no rhythm), cycling (not a fan—her knees and bottom hurt), spinning (it took a while, but she found the right way to sit in the saddle and now she's fully into it), running (in her repertoire now, too), and CrossFit. CrossFit, if you haven't heard of it yet, is a combination of interval training, resistance training, kettle bell lifting, plyometrics, gymnastics, and a few other strongman-type activities. All our cast members on *Extreme Weight Loss* do it three to four times a week, and it is *hard*. Yet you think you can never be a CrossFit enthusiast and one day, like Amber, you're dead-lifting 280 pounds and you're hooked. (Just for the record, I am not personally a fan of CrossFit. I love the sense of community and how passionate its devotees are, but I hate the fact that people are encouraged to dead-lift heavy weights when they're in a state of severe fatigue. We make sure our cast members use caution when they're doing CrossFit workouts, and I advise you, if you try them, to do the same.)

The transformation of attitude toward exercise we see is astounding. Cast members even get to the point where they see doing the "wall wash" as a point of pride. This is a phenomenon, so named by the Season 1 contestants of *The Biggest Loser*, where your arms are so sore from exercise the day before that you can't even lift them up to scrub your hair so you squirt the shampoo against the wall and rub your head on it. This is no joke. Washing your hair becomes hard work.

Once upon a time, you were a little kid who loved to run around. With very few exceptions, we all did. Go back and find that feeling again. Also, think about all of the things you have survived in your life. It doesn't have to be a big trauma, but everybody has stuff. Maybe you went through a tough breakup or divorce. Someone you loved died. You failed a class in school. A friend betrayed you. You got fired. And you survived. In all of those instances, you figured out a way to not end up in a dark room forever suffering from that pain. You moved on. Mentally, you are already strong. Use that strength to power you through your workouts.

Exercising when you are fat is doubly hard. I'm aware of that.

The more weight you have, the harder it is to move. To give you a sense of it, grab two 20-pound dumbbells, and go for a 10-minute run on the treadmill. Then, put them down and do it again. See what a difference just carrying an extra 40 pounds makes? It's nearly impossible to run 10 minutes! (One the other hand, failing at this little exercise gives you a sense of how much easier moving around will be if you *lose* 40 pounds.)

That is not all you're up against if you're carrying a lot of extra weight. There is also the awful feeling of having to walk into a gym and feel like the fat person. Panda felt so embarrassed that he joined a 24-hour gym so he could go in the wee hours when nobody was there. It was the only time he felt comfortable working out. Not ideal, but the point is that he found a way to do it. Going to the gym late at night helped him lose about 50 pounds before he even came on the show. Maybe for you it's exercising in a welcoming environment. Many women gravitate to Zumba and other types of dance classes for just that reason.

For the most part, weight loss is simple math. Newer research suggests that a calorie is not always a calorie—in other words, some calories are more fattening than others. But for our purposes let's stick to a formula that may be imperfect but gives you a ballpark figure to work with: calories eaten minus calories burned equals pounds lost. Every 3,500 calories of deficit is equal to about 1 pound of weight loss. So if you eat 2,000 calories and burn 3,000 a day for seven days you will lose about 2 pounds per week. Don't freak out—you don't have to burn 3,000 calories on the treadmill every day. Your body burns calories all day long even if you do nothing but lie in bed, so the 3,000 I'm asking you to burn includes that freebie.

You're probably wondering how many freebie calories a day you get. It's different for different people and at different times. Some people have a higher metabolism than others, plus the percentage of body fat you carry as well as both your internal and the external (read: weather) temperature can figure into the equation. To get a close estimate, search the Internet for a Basal Metabolic Rate (BMR) or Mifflin-St Jeor formula. Either one will help you calculate your resting calorie burn off.

The 3,000 calories a day I mentioned, even if they include that gift of calories at rest, may still be too much for you to fit into your life, but come on! At least try for 500 beyond your at-rest number. You're in the losing phase, so you're going to need to do extra. And the 500 I am asking for will help bump up your body's metabolism, giving you the "extra burn" you always hear about. When you hit the stage where you're maintaining rather than losing weight, you can ramp it down a bit. At all stages, set a goal that feels reachable . . . then go a little beyond. For instance, set your watch to run 30 minutes, but then stretch it to 35. Make your body listen to your brain! Get that burn in, and soon you'll crave it.

Speaking of maintenance, it is very, very hard to maintain weight loss without exercise. James O. Hill, PhD, who is the founding executive director of the Anschutz Health and Wellness Center at the University of Colorado Anschutz Medical Campus where we hold the *Extreme Weight Loss* Boot Camps, also happens to be the co-founder of the National Weight Control Registry. The Registry, which has been joined by more than 6,000 people who have lost weight and kept it off, has allowed researchers to study what all those successful people have in common. One thing the registry has shown is that people who maintain their weight after shedding pounds share a devotion to exercise. The overwhelming majority of the participants in the study (89 percent) combined diet and exercise to lose weight, and Dr. Hill calls exercise one of the best predictors of who's going to keep the weight off. More than half of those maintainers do about 3 hours of exercise per week (I, of course, say do more!) You'd be crazy not to add exercise into the mix. It not only helps you lose weight, but it makes you feel good. I have never regretted doing a workout. Yes, your muscles may ache when you're just starting out, but I think most people would agree that it's a good kind of ache. It's a badge of honor.

So when I wake up in the dark, and don't really want to get out of bed, I tell myself that after it is over, I know I will feel good for doing it, and if I don't do it, I will feel guilty all day! That gets me moving. But if you need more motivation, try to create a streak. Can you avoid hitting the snooze button for 20 straight days? Be proud of each day you keep the streak alive. Brag about it to let people know that you aren't kidding.

You might remember that, before she slimmed down, got that convertible, and turned into an exercise adventurer, Elaine was a typical yo-yoer. She'd get fat, she'd get skinny. Repeat. At one point, she'd lost about 40 pounds and thought to herself, *I know how to diet, but exercise is missing.* It wasn't as though she'd never tried. She had; it just never took. But Elaine knew she had to do it, even if she didn't really want to. So she called a friend who was in good shape and asked her to recommend a trainer. She made an appointment.

Most people would go to their first meeting with a fitness trainer and put on a good face. They'll usually say stuff like, "Let's do it!" "I'm excited to get started!" Not Elaine. "In my heart, I knew I had to tell him the truth," she says, "so I said, 'I will show up on day one with the best intentions, then a few days later, I'll text or email some BS excuse of why I can't come to the next session. Slowly, ever so slowly, I will disappear on you. I don't believe this will work, but I'm here.' "

This sounds like a classic case of the person who says "I can't" and is right. But Elaine had the good fortune to be talking to someone who got her and welcomed her honesty. He helped her modify exercises to accommodate the orthopedic challenges she had because her weight put so much pressure on her joints, and contrary to what Elaine expected, he didn't think she was a loser because she could only do 3 minutes on the elliptical trainer. He made a safe place for her, loved her, and believed in her. And as a result, she thrived. She climbed that hill in Jerusalem, she bought new clothes, she stayed the course.

That trainer's name is Steve Mareska, and he is one of the most motivating fitness professionals I have ever known. He creates the temple, church, place of worship—a safe place—instead of trying to motivate through fear. Steve not only opens his doors to his clients but also he opens his heart (I know because I work out with him, too.) To impress him is to impress your rabbi or priest. Go find yourself a Steve, and you will never *not* want to be in shape again. I always leave his place of "worship" filled up emotionally and worn down physically. I love going there, and it might sound silly, but that hour I spend with him sets me up for success the entire day.

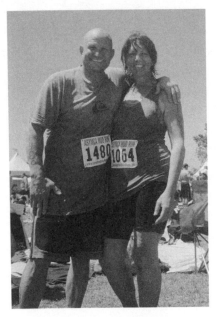

Elaine with her trainer, Steve

One day in the gym, Elaine saw some guys hitting a heavy punching bag (one of those guys was me). "That looks cool," she thought, but she didn't want to try it. "I thought I might hurt myself." Steve convinced her to give it a go, and it triggered a revelation. "I never knew how much rage I had inside me," says Elaine. "I'd wail on that bag, and it would all come out. It was such a gift. A healthy way to get it out rather than stuffing food down my throat."

Okay, so what's the upshot here? One, find people who will help you see the light. It doesn't have to be a trainer; not everyone can afford that. You might, though, be able to pay for a few sessions just to have someone show you the right things to do in a gym. Don't let fear of making a fool of yourself in the gym stop you. Even Robert and Raymond, who had played sports in high school, felt at a loss of what to do whenever they went to a gym. Find that friend or relative who loves exercise, and let them take you under their wing. Join a group. Start a group. Unless you are really self-disciplined (and my guess is you're not), don't just buy a workout DVD and try to exercise in front of your TV at home. You're never going to do it. Get out there with people who will hold you accountable, expect you to show up, introduce you to new ways to move your body, and keep you company. Find your exercise community.

When Amber went home after Boot Camp, she was determined to change her social relationships—relationships that had previously been built around going out for burgers, meeting for frozen mocha drinks, maybe taking in a movie (and a large-size bucket of popcorn). Now she wanted to build her relationships around exercise. Here's how she did it: She started signing up for fun runs and posting her plans on Facebook. "Hey, this week I'm doing the 5K down at the beach, anyone interested?" She'd then take note of who said they might join her, write it down in her datebook, and call them to follow up. "Let's do it," she'd say. "Even if we're the only two people in our group of friends, let's do it!" Like Amber, be the recruiter. Take on the responsibility of making others accountable to you. That will also ensure the reverse—that you will have to be accountable to *them*.

Moving connects you to people, which is why we are on this Earth! Connection feeds the soul, and for a lot less calories then a triple-fudge sundae. A sundae lasts about 5 minutes; human connections can last a lifetime. **There are billions of people on the planet . . . go experience some of them.**

Here's the other thing to be learned from Elaine's experience, Amber's, too. Exercise is the best antidepressant in the world. If everyone would do it, the pharmaceutical industry would be out of business! Forget your co-pay, and make exercise your coping go-to. If you're angry, hit it, run it out, or walk it out. If you're stressed, hop on your bike, hike up a hill. If you're sad, get into the gym and start lifting weights or take a cardio class. There's no better way to take your mind off what ails you than having to concentrate on not dropping a weight or crashing into the person next to you during Zumba.

From now on, the treadmill is your Prozac. I guarantee that you will feel better after you exercise—and so much better than if you were drowning your sorrows in plates of macaroni and cheese. Not only are there tons of studies that show that exercise is an effective antidote to depression but also there is some research to suggest that comfort foods aren't really even that comforting. In a study at the University of Minnesota, the researchers induced a bad mood in people and found that those in a group that ate foods like brownies and apple pie to soothe themselves didn't perk up any more than the group that ate healthy foods or nothing at all.

Here's the thing. Eating comfort food is only comforting for a short time. Then you just feel miserable; **comfort food always comes with a side of remorse.** But exercise doesn't. Have you ever met anyone who felt guilty for spending an hour swimming laps or working out on a stationary bike? No one comes out of a spinning class and says, "Oops, I shouldn't have done that." No, instead we feel great when we move. Movement is incredibly more soothing than food.

Something exercise-related you should remember (I've said this before but it bears repeating here): Don't reward yourself for a hard workout with food that isn't good for you. So many people will say, "Oh, I worked out so hard, this piece of cake is my reward." Reward? Never reward doing something right with doing something wrong. Instead, reward right with right—something like a nutritionally dense, healthy lunch that will keep your metabolism humming at its highest levels. Or treat yourself to a new piece of exercise gear or clothing. Reward yourself by taking your pants to a tailor and getting them taken in. Buy a new pair of shoes. Choose something that will make you feel good in the long run versus something like a cupcake, which will only feel good while you're eating it. This may not be such a difficult adjustment. Once you start caring for your body in one way, it can inspire you to care for your body in other ways. Eating healthfully will come naturally.

CHAPTER 17

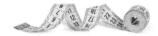

Do the Impossible

If you've been sitting on your butt every day for the past fifteen years, just getting to the point where you exercise every day is a pretty amazing feat. But what if you did something *really* amazing, so amazing that no one, least of all you, believed you were capable of it? It would rock your world.

I've seen hundreds of people do the seemingly impossible, from running marathons after never running more than a mile in their lives, to climbing up the stairs of a 100-story building after struggling to walk up the flight of stairs at home just to get into bed. Each season, we ask our cast members to do something extremely challenging, but nothing is as demanding as the 7,000-calorie-burn challenge. That's when we ask the cast to burn 7,000 calories in *one* day. The calories they burn just through the daily process of living and breathing doesn't count. The 7,000 calories have to all be burned through exercise. And let me give you a sense of how much energy you have to put into it: Running a marathon burns approximately 3,500 calories, so the 7,000-calorie challenge is equivalent to the energy it would take to run two full marathons in one day!

There's absolutely *no* good physiological reason in the world to burn 7,000 calories in one day, but it delivers an incredible psychological payoff. A lot of the people we work with on our shows think that everything is impossible. "I'm not a runner, I can't run." "I can't get a job." "I can't lose weight." For them to accomplish something so ridiculous that they and everybody else think it's impossible, well, it becomes a badge of honor. It gives them a new perspective on themselves and their lives. That's what I see it offering to you as well. As I've said in earlier chapters, there's great value in small victories and small changes. But if you can handle it (and anyone who puts his or her mind to it can), doing something drastic can speed up the process of change. And by the way, after you've done something like the 7,000-calorie burn, the next time someone asks you to burn 2,000 calories in a day (let alone just go to the gym for an hour's workout), you're going to say, "I can do that before breakfast!"

My favorite 7,000-calorie-burn story belongs to a cast member from *The Revolution*. Jen was single mom who'd recently recovered from a rare form of cancer. She had a hysterectomy because of the cancer, and afterward put on a lot of weight. Her son, Ryan, who was ten at the time, loved *The Biggest Loser*. He printed out an application, filled it out, and brought it to her. It was her wake-up call. "I thought, Oh God, I'd better do something about the weight I've gained," says Jen. So she and Ryan made a video, sent it in, and were contacted by our staff—not for *The Biggest Loser*, but for *The Revolution*.

Like *Extreme Weight Loss*, *The Revolution* sent cast members to Boot Camp. One day, I made them an offer: The first person who can burn 7,000 calories in one day will win an iPad. One woman said she'd do it that weekend. Then Jen chimed in. "I have a competitiveness in me from being an athlete in high school, and I wanted to win that iPad for my son," she remembers. "I couldn't afford to buy one."

||||||||||||||||||||||||||||||||||||||||||||||||||||||||||||||||||||||||||||

One Challenge Leads to Another

JD,

On Thursday, my "comrades in arms," Derik and Brian, and I all decided to take on the epic 7,000-calorie challenge you gave us. We all had a lot of random commitments throughout the day (filming, work, etc.), but we didn't let that stop us! We *all* completed it!

I did mine split up between a total of 5 workouts for a total of 10.5 hours! The last 2 hours really sucked at first, but as the trainer Joey reminded me, this day was a marathon not a sprint. And ironically, that's exactly what I did. On Thursday, I logged over 27.2 miles! No wonder I felt so tired and spent—I did an entire marathon!

However, I felt euphoric and rejuvenated at the end! I am already looking for the next challenge.

—Cheyanne, Fat Chance cast member, via email

Jen—and Ryan, who stayed with her the whole day, working out with her part of the time and cheerleading the rest—hit the gym first thing in the morning. And by first thing, I mean at dawn. They took spin classes, worked out on the treadmill, rowing machine, and the stair-climber, moving from machine to machine, hour after hour. And that was just the warm-up! They didn't stop. Another one of the women who'd taken on the challenge (and the one Jen saw as her nemesis in this particular competition) was going just as hard; she and Jen were neck and neck the whole day, posting the developments online as they went even though they were doing it in different states. (To keep track of their progress—and keep them honest—we had given them FitBits, wearable computers that calculate how many calories you're burning.) "We have to beat her!" Jen told Ryan. When Jen had about 500 calories more to go, after nearly 20 straight hours of working out, the gym announced that it would be closing in twenty minutes. It was already ten o'clock at night, and they'd noticed that Jen's rival had stopped posting her progress. So what did they do? Call it a day? Say, "I *almost* made it to 7,000"? No way. There is no special T-shirt for almost finishing something. Inspired by how close they were to completing the impossible, they went outside and ran around the gym by the light of the moon. "Every time we'd pass this one corner we could see bats, but we kept going," says Jen. "I don't know what came over me that night. Up until then, I had only exercised one hour, sometimes two hours a day, but I didn't want to let my son down. I wanted to prove to myself that I could do it, too."

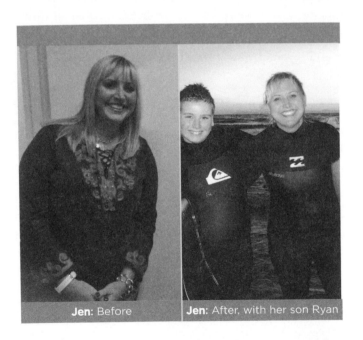

Jen: Before   **Jen:** After, with her son Ryan

Needless to say, Jen won the iPad for Ryan. But that was really the least of what she gave her son that day. His mom had just shown him how powerful she was. She wasn't the sick incapacitated person who was going to die from cancer; she was a force of nature, a superhero. That kid (who's now a high-school football player with offers for a full college scholarship) will never forget the night his mom did the impossible. She taught him that a person can do anything he puts his mind to. Jen taught herself that lesson, too. "Every day, on my way to work, I drive by that corner where we'd see the bats and smile," she says. "That was the day I realized that your mind is in control of your body. You can convince yourself to do anything." So, yeah, no real physical advantage to burning 7,000 calories in one day, but 7,000 reasons to do it and prove to you and your family that you are special. You can achieve anything if you want it badly enough. Quitting is always easier. So is choosing a cupcake over a bowl of broccoli. But if you start making the herculean tasks normal choices, they become much easier.

We get a fair amount of criticism for asking the people on our shows to test their limits in a big way. It's true that we often ask them to do things they hate or are afraid of, things they think are impossible, but I firmly believe the payoff is worth it. And the feedback we get is priceless. "When we triumph, we have a victory, and all of the sudden our posture is higher and we're smiling more," says Jennifer, the *Extreme Weight Loss* cast member I told you about in Chapter 4. "I don't slouch anymore, and I smile. That might seem like a minor thing, but I used to slump over and frown, and I never smiled. It's because of those victories."

The last time I spoke to Vanessa, a cast member on a show of ours called *Fat Chance,* she was getting ready to take off to Paris and Barcelona. Her career was taking off big time, too, and she believes completing the 7,000-calorie-burn challenge played a role in how things are going. "After I did the challenge, I thought to myself, 'If I can do this, I can do anything,'" says Vanessa.

Vanessa came on the show weighing in at 235 and hoping to lose 100 pounds. Her problem was the age-old food-as-a-coping mechanism syndrome. Anytime things got rough, Vanessa ate—

and ate and ate. But now, here she was on the show, losing weight at a good but not great pace and still needing to go further, when I challenged the *Fat Chance* group to do something spectacular, something bigger than they ever thought they could do. Vanessa immediately got fired up—only her trainer said she didn't think Vanessa could do it. That was all she had to hear. Vanessa took care of the obligations she had that day, including her regular workout (which put her ahead of the game), then went straight to the gym armed with protein bars and other snacks to keep her going over what she knew was going to be a long haul. At 8:00 p.m., just as the summer sun was setting, she began her mission to prove that trainer wrong, and she didn't stop until the sun came up. "I left the gym at 6:17 the next morning," says Vanessa, who burned the calories by alternating sessions on different exercise machines with fuel breaks in between.

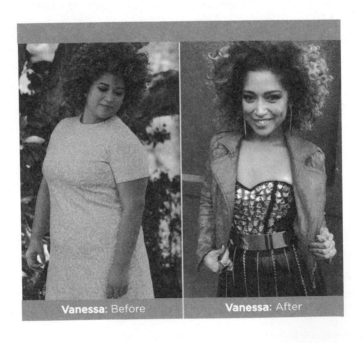

Vanessa: Before   **Vanessa**: After

||||||||||||||||||||||||||||||||||||||||||||||||||||||||||||||||||||||||||||||||

Finding the Strength That Lives in You

Hi JD,

This challenge was one of the scariest, most seemingly impossible, and altering moments of my life. I really had to face myself in the final hours . . . and I realized I have someone to be proud of whispering in my ear to keep going, to fight, to overcome, and to finish strong. That person was me. And as crazy it sounds, that realization gave me a sense of respect for myself that I haven't felt in a long time . . . or ever. Your challenge was a gift. Thank you JD!

—Vanessa, *Fat Chance* cast member, via email

I loved reading the notes she kept as she went along (see page 194) because it shows what a roller-coaster ride tackling a big challenge is, as well as how Vanessa toughed it out even when she thought she couldn't take another step. At times she felt dismal; she even broke down and cried a few times. "Body starting to shut down. Mind wants to keep going. It's too late to stop now," Vanessa wrote with 3,018 calories to go. With 1,181 left: "I can't seem to move—the edge I found for the big push seems to be fading. I think 2 hours left. Just don't think about it." And she kept going! Then, not only did she finish, she mastered something that will help her achieve every goal she sets. "Your mind can be your biggest ally or your biggest enemy," says Vanessa. "I learned how to tell it to shut up."

Think about taking on a big challenge this way: Your body absolutely has the ability to do it; it's your mind-set you've got to contend with. But you can do that! You're in control of your own brain!

Here is a good way to do a big calorie burn even if you don't have a way of calculating your calories: Find out what time the sun rises in your area, get up a few minutes before, get ready, pack water, a sandwich and some snacks, and start walking. And don't stop until the sun sets. Figure out how long the day is going to be (just Google the sunrise and sunset times in your area for the day),

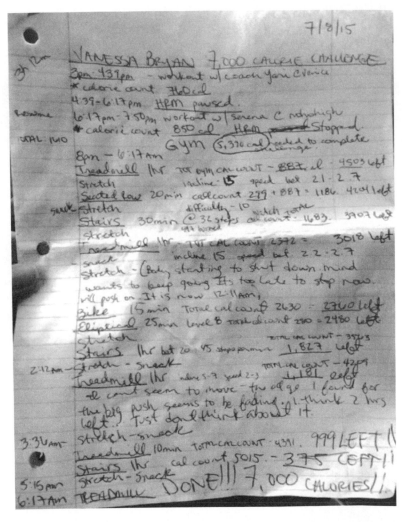

Vanessa's notes from her 7,000-calorie challenge

then decide on a reasonable turnaround point. Bear in mind that you may start by walking at three miles per hour, but by the time you're near the end, you may be moving closer to one mile per hour. There's no exact science here; just calculate the best you can. Bring a phone so that if you get stuck far from home, you can call a friend to come get you.

The whole purpose of this is to push yourself to a point you never thought possible. Do you have to train for it? Not really. Sure, people train for a whole year before they do a marathon, but our experience tells me that even people who have only been working out for a little while can do an immense challenge. The cast members on *The Revolution* who did the 7,000-calorie burn had only been working out for a month before they took on the challenge. It's your head, not your body, that drives you to finish, so that's what you really have to get in shape—your brain. Believe you can do it, and you will. Do people stop and take a break? Sure (mostly to cry!), but by the end of the burn, they're so empowered that they feel like they could keep going for another 24 hours. Probably the hardest thing about doing a serious challenge is the angst leading up to it. So if you decide to do something extreme, don't wait long—each day you wait is just another stomach-churning load of anxiety. When someone says, "Oh I have a headache, I don't think I should do it today. I'll do it tomorrow," I always say, "Okay, but you're just giving yourself another day of fear and worry. Just do it, and be done with it."

As with anything, it can help to have company. On *The Revolution*, there were about 12 out of 15 people who said they were going to do the 7,000-calorie challenge. "Yeah, we're going to text each other every hour and send pics, all at the same time." Eventually, the other three caved. "Okay, we'll do it, too." It was a positive kind of peer pressure, and those last-minute joiners were the happiest of all when the whole thing was over. I've never heard someone finish and say, "I wish I hadn't done that." It's always the greatest accomplishment of their lives! And it really cements change. Who's going to cheat the next day after completing such a feat? Once you start stacking accomplishments on top of each other, and the stack gets higher and higher, it makes the wall that you've built up around you—the one that's keeping you from making positive change—get lower and lower.

One of the odd things about doing a 7,000-calorie challenge is that it doesn't really help you lose weight in the short term. It seems like you'd lose at least two pounds (remember 3,500 is about equal to a pound), and some people do; however, the stress of the effort also kicks the body into survival mode. "Oh my God, what are you doing to me?" your body will ask, then it will slow your metabolism for the next few days. This is nothing to worry about; your calorie burning will go back to normal. But this challenge is really about changing your mind, not your body. Once you do it, you'll know you're totally up to the task of eating healthfully and exercising regularly. That will be a piece of cake!

CHAPTER 18

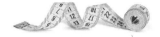

Make Mistakes—Then Move On

You know how it goes. You go to a party, drink too much, start dipping into the chips and guacamole, and the next thing you know, you're on your way home having eaten the macaroni and cheese and a big hunk of birthday cake. The next day, instead of having your oatmeal or smoothie for breakfast, you say what the heck and stop at Bob's Doughnuts on the way to work. From there, it's just a slow slide into debauchery.

You've heard it a million times: Everyone makes mistakes. You're going to screw up, eat too much, slack off on exercise. It's inevitable. Occasional failure is part of the process. But the fact that you make mistakes is not what defines you. **What defines you is what you do after you make mistakes.** Do you beat yourself up, get emotional about it, then send yourself into a pizza-and-potato-chip-eating spiral? Most fat people do; that's often why they're fat.

Never hold a mistake against yourself. That's pure self-sabotage. It turns into a self-defeating cycle. You cheat, get angry with yourself, then decide that you don't deserve to be fit and healthy— you're just a loser. What sets the people who lose weight and keep it off apart from those who don't is that they don't freak out and punish themselves every time they eat something they shouldn't.

They acknowledge that they've screwed up; then they *move on*. Moving on is key. Get back on the horse. Immediately. Nobody is perfect, and you shouldn't expect yourself to be. Don't think of mistakes as evidence that you have no willpower. After all, you're only one meal away from getting back to healthy eating. One day of unhealthy eating never made anyone fat. But the emotional weight of thinking you can't handle the challenge because you had one bad day *will* make you fat. Give yourself a break. If one bad choice is the end of your effort, what does that say about you? Do you quit everything as soon as one thing goes badly? Find the grit to stay with it. After making a bad choice, choose to consciously make two good ones. That will put you one choice ahead of the game.

|||||||||||||||||||||||||||||||||||||||||||||||||||||||||||||||||||||||||

Coping with Ups and Downs

Here are my biggest takeaways: Begin each day with the end (your goals) in mind! It's okay to fail, but it's not okay to be a failure! Continue to decide how much the rest of your life is worth, and move ahead accordingly! Inspiration starts within!

—Stacey, posted on *The Revolution* Facebook page

In my experience, you'll be less likely to make mistakes in the first place if you recast your own image of yourself. Just like vegetarians don't eat meat, people who want to exist at a healthy weight don't eat lots of junky food. It's against their self-imposed rules. During *Extreme Weight Loss*'s Boot Camp, there's a tradition of giving cast members a fun day (also known as a cheat day). That's a day where they're allowed to cheat without us getting on their cases. I let it go because I believe so much in the ability of Chris

Powell, the host and head trainer on *Extreme Weight Loss,* to get weight off people, but I don't agree with him on this one. We have actually had many discussions over this issue, and it's the one thing we can't see eye-to-eye on. I think the ideal is to have small indulgences and work them into your regular routine. A cookie here. An ice-cream cone there. Maybe a small bag of chips once in a while. It's just part of your lifestyle. Instead, the fun day implies that you deprive yourself for six days, then on the seventh think, "Oh man, am I going to open up and have whatever I want." That's just a bad habit to get into. Because, suddenly, your one fun day bleeds into a second fun day, then a third, and pretty soon, you're back where you started. Or maybe you approach it by going hog-wild on your fun day and then cutting back severely the next day as penance. Then you're essentially bingeing and purging, which is not at all healthy.

There's also evidence that ping-ponging between "good" and "bad" eating is not conducive to keeping weight off. One study by the National Weight Loss Registry researchers looked at who better maintained weight loss: people who consistently maintained their diet throughout the week or people who loosened up over the weekend then went back to healthy eating during the week. Not surprisingly (to me, at least), the consistent people were 1.5 times more likely to keep the pounds off.

As the registry researchers discovered, weekends off can be a slippery slope; I'd say the same goes for the weekly "fun day." But let's say that you do decide to have your own "fun day," and it starts bleeding into the following day. When you make a mistake, tell somebody. Call up a friend on the phone, and talk about it. Just putting it out there can be incredibly liberating. You'll find it easier to just move on. Otherwise, you're going to plant your butt on the couch with a carton of ice cream and wallow in shame and self-pity.

Another way to avoid wallowing is to look at obstacles as inspirations. You can either be tortured and depressed by your slip-ups, or inspired by them. Try to figure out what made you stray from your promises to yourself and take preventive actions so it doesn't happen again. There's always a solution if you want to find it.

A few years ago, my oldest son got the most difficult teacher in the whole school, Mr. Rucker. Everyone felt threatened by the guy; he intimidates the entire student body. Why? Because he expects his students to give their best every day. And if they don't, he will hold them accountable. He gives three big tests throughout the year called the pebble, the rock, and the boulder. The boulder is the hardest test given by any teacher in the entire school. When my son came home upset about getting Mr. Rucker, I said to him, "You know, you can go along with everyone else who is scared of this guy, or you can look at this guy and find out what makes him tick. What does he have to offer you?"

Mr. Rucker obviously loves to teach and he is passionate about preparing kids for the future. But he makes them earn their grade. Getting an "A" in Mr. Rucker's class is the equivalent to getting a compliment from Jillian Michaels, the hard-driving trainer on *The Biggest Loser*. It is earned. Turns out, my son now considers this scary guy his favorite teacher of all time. And he's learned more from Mr. Rucker than from any other teacher he's had. By reframing the way he looked at the teacher from the beginning, he overcame what could have been a formidable obstacle. "Look at the experience you've had," I told him, "You'll never forget the guy." That is truly looking at an obstacle and turning it into an inspiration. By the way, he got an "A" in the class. He kicked that boulder's ass, and I am so very proud of him.

One thing you are never going to be able to avoid, no matter how virtuous you are, is temptation. Temptation is always going to be there. You can't make it go away. But you can be mindful. Think about whether you want to waste your calories on something that really isn't that great. Ask yourself if you are really hungry, or if you're just eating to fill time or because you're stressed. You can have your two minutes of comfort or however long it's going to take you to plow through a burger and fries, but once the food is gone, your problem will likely still be there. And you've just topped it off with a giant scoop of guilt.

Rules to Live By

Hi You Guys,

The fact is, if you do our program, if you exercise and eat clean, you lose weight. The pounds drop. If you don't? You gain 13 pounds in two weeks. So:

- Don't eat steak except flank steak at 9 p.m.
- Drink your allotted water.
- Don't buy premade ANYTHING. Go to the store (like I did yesterday) and shop how we know how to shop.
- Don't go to a restaurant, even a Village Inn, without checking their online menu first.
- Eat more than one or two meals for the entire day.
- GET REST! EIGHT HOURS OR MORE IS ESSENTIAL!
- Don't EVER rest on your laurels and maybe sorta, kinda think you are invincible or that you can never gain because you haven't.
- Don't allow the stress of the day to get you down.

But most important?

If you do any of these things (and I did them all) DON'T ALLOW THE MISTAKES AND SETBACKS AND ADVERSITY TO DEFEAT YOU!

—Rod, *Extreme Weight Loss* cast member, via email

You will make mistakes; everyone does. But put some strategic plans in place to make it harder to make mistakes. At my house dinner can be a trying time. We have two boys who are "sta-a-a-a-arving" all the time. My wife doesn't want to just feed them anything; she wants to make healthy, complete meals. But each person in the family also has a certain way they want their food prepared. As I said, it's a trying time. So we developed a trick to prime the boys for healthy eating that has worked so well that, if we don't do it, they now ask for it. About 30 minutes before dinnertime, we invite the kids to the dinner table to do homework. As they sit there, they can smell what's cooking and hear the sizzle of the pans. This starts their little mouths to watering and gets them even hungrier. We all know that feeling—at that point, you'd eat a chair if it was covered in vanilla icing. Now that we have them in our clutches, we cut up red peppers, Persian cucumbers, and carrots and stack them high on a plate. As they're doing their homework, smelling the food, and getting hungrier by the minute, they just start blindly grabbing the veggies. It's as if we'd served them Double-Stuf Oreos. Most times, they argue over who gets the last red pepper. So what have we accomplished? We have gotten our kids to eat nutrient-dense food that they might have otherwise shunned, and primed them for the healthy dinner to come.

You can do this for yourself, too. Put healthy food in your way, and you'll eat it. It will fill you up, and you'll be less likely to get caught with your hand in the cookie jar.

Make it easy for you to succeed. Talking yourself down can help, too. Say out loud, "I am better than this (insert tempting food here)," or give yourself a mantra (see page 232) to deal with temptation. Or, maybe you do something physical. Every time you feel tempted to cut yourself a slice of cake or unwrap a candy bar, do ten push-ups. By the end of the day, you could be 200 push-ups in before you realize your arms are too sore to pick up the cake anyway.

When all else fails and you indulge anyway, figure out how many calories you ate, then burn triple that number of calories on the treadmill that day. No waiting, no avoiding. You eat a bite of cheesecake, and it's 50 calories? Great. Go burn 150 calories running up and down your stairs at home. Every decision you make in life has a consequence, and the sooner you deal with it, the less likely you will be to continue to let it happen. Pretty soon, you will do the math *before* you order that double chocolate-chip frappe and realize it ain't worth it! You are worth more!

CHAPTER 19

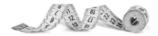

Keep the Pounds from Coming Back

If you don't want to gain back the weight you've lost, keep doing what you're doing. It's as simple as that. Don't backtrack. This is obviously easier said than done because, within the general population, most people who lose weight *do* gain it back. The statistics vary, but it's somewhere in the neighborhood of 65 percent of people gain back the weight they lose after a year; 95 percent gain it all back after three years. Pretty dismal. Our shows have a far better success rate: 65 percent of people on all our shows keep the weight off *permanently* (we've been tracking them since 2004). Every once in a while, though, a former cast member reaches out to me to say they've slipped up in a big way.

Anyone who's lost weight can gain it back, even the people who did it on TV. That's why you have to stay on guard—and nobody likes to hear this—for the rest of your life. This doesn't mean you can never have a slice of pizza or take a day off from exercise, but as you surely know by now, you can't think of it in terms of "I went on a diet, I lost weight, and now I can go back to normal!" You now have a new normal. Everything you did to lose weight is normal for you now. And the life you were living before was *not* normal, or you wouldn't have ended up as large as you did. You didn't know what normal looked like. Now you do.

I think it's helpful to know what went wrong with people who gained back weight. What can you learn from their mistakes? One former contestant I've stayed in touch with is Ashley, who lost 183 pounds on *The Biggest Loser* (and gained a fiancé, one of the other contestants, in the process). Ashley came on with her mom (the two of them always wore pink) and proceeded to lose about 49 percent of her body weight, an amazing feat, by anyone's standards. Yet she put back on a lot of the pounds a few years later. Okay, more then a lot. She lost 183 pounds . . . and gained back 185.

Ashley, who has since gotten back on track (you can see some of her emails to me scattered throughout this book), is very clear-eyed about what happened. For one thing, she let fear get the best of her, and it became a self-fulfilling prophecy. "I was so afraid of gaining back the weight that I weighed myself six times a day," says Ashley. "Then my body listened to my brain, and after six months, I *did* gain the pounds back."

||||||||||||||||||||||||||||||||||||||||||||||||||||||||||||||||||||||||||||||||

You Know What to Do—Now Do It!

Good Morning JD!

I hope you and your family are well! When I applied for *The Biggest Loser*, one of my main goals was to be able to lose the weight so I could start a family. Little Ethan is now 9 weeks old, and I could not be happier!

Before going on *The Biggest Loser*, I would have said things like "I have tried *everything* to lose weight." "Nothing has worked." "If I only knew the right way." Truth be told, those of us who have tried "everything" to lose weight know a lot more than we give ourselves credit for.

—Kristin, *The Biggest Loser* contestant, via email

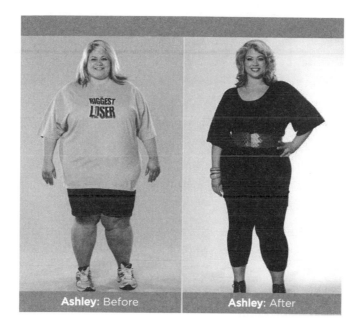

Ashley: Before   Ashley: After

Obviously, she didn't just imagine the pounds coming back on, and they magically appeared; but her fear and obsession with the scale made it difficult to feel confident and empowered. She lost sight of all the hurdles she'd overcome and started to beat herself up every time she made a mistake. In her misery, she reverted to the old habits that got her on *The Biggest Loser* in the first place. It was hard to get out of bed in the morning—let alone make it to a workout.

There's also more to the story. "I strongly believe that weight loss is more of a mental than a physical battle," says Ashley, "and I still had things I hadn't dealt with. My unresolved issues were awoken working with trainers Jillian Michaels and Bob Harper on *The Biggest Loser*, but it's like an onion with several layers—you need to remove them one by one until you get to the core. I thought that I was fixed after six months, but it took me 29 years to get where I was, so I can see now that it does take time."

It's not going to surprise you to hear me say this: Your state of mind is everything. It's key to keeping the weight off. Dealing with your issues. Believing in yourself. Both of those things are critical. There's a young guy named Josh who made it to the finals week of *Extreme Weight Loss,* but ultimately didn't make it on the show— yet went on to lose 308 pounds on his own and kept the weight off. His experience was completely different from Ashley's, and I wondered what accounted for his success.

When Josh tried out for the show, he was 28 years old and close to 600 pounds (he's 6'9", so he can carry a lot more weight than most people, but still that was dangerous). He told me that he lost 26 pounds during finals week, and it helped him realize that he didn't need a show to get the weight off. "I was sick of making excuses for myself," he says, "and I started to believe that I could do it." That last part—believing in himself—was what really turned his life around.

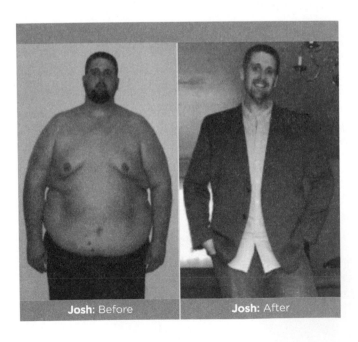

Josh: Before   Josh: After

For a long time, Josh had been unhappy with how unhealthy he'd become, though he kept up the façade that all was good with his life—even though he didn't attend his own college graduation because he didn't want to deal with a cap and gown that didn't fit. Josh was very social and a partier, so when he resolved to change his body, he had to change just about everything in his life. He gave himself a year, stopped going out to bars and started living a quieter life. "I thought to myself, 'If my friends don't understand, then they're not really my friends.'" Turns out, they supported him big time, and as he got more comfortable with his new lifestyle, he started going places again—but doing it his way, bringing a cooler with healthy food and a big jug of water to cookouts, for instance, so he could eat and drink the way he wanted. He put control into his own hands, which is so empowering. What all this did was feed Josh's confidence. "So many people don't believe in themselves. When I discovered that I wasn't just physically strong, but mentally and emotionally strong, that's when I hit my stride."

I love this story because not only does it show that you don't need a reality show to lose large amounts of weight, but it highlights the importance of looking at your accomplishments and using them to keep pushing you forward—and prevent you from falling back. Think about why you've done this, and how much you've achieved. Don't focus on what the scale says. If you become obsessed with the number like Ashley did, the weight is going to come right back on. Come back to your purpose, and think about the mental and emotional hurdles you have overcome. It doesn't matter if those hurdles seem relatively small ("I always thought I hated running") or large ("I finally got help to deal with the abuse that happened to me years ago"); keep them in mind. Why did you do this? How far have you come?

There are also some practical things you can do to keep from regaining the weight you've lost. One thing former cast member and current *Extreme Weight Loss* trainer Bruce said he learned along the way was that a lot of people try to figure out a new way to eat instead of sticking with the diet that helped them lose in the first place. Don't change it up. Stick with what helped you be successful. "Don't think, 'I can probably tweak it here and tweak it there,'" he says. "Stay with what got you where you are."

But, as you keep your dietary practices fixed, don't be complacent about what you do and don't know. Keep educating yourself on the finer points of healthy living. "There were so many things I didn't know in the beginning," says Bruce. "I didn't know what a carb was. I didn't know that a fresh chicken breast has only 75 milligrams of sodium versus the frozen packaged ones, which have 360 milligrams. I didn't know that a russet potato has more calories than a red potato. I didn't realize how many vegetables there are and how you can make them taste good. I didn't know I could love mushrooms, onions, and peppers. I never thought I'd sit down to eat a pepper like an apple and enjoy it. I feel as though I learn something helpful every week. You have to be a lifelong learner."

One thing that almost everyone says after they've changed their eating and exercise habits is that they feel a lot better. Don't lose sight of how good you feel when you're exercising regularly and eating well. That was crucial in Robert and Raymond's transformation. "We're actually feeling energy from the foods we take in; we can feel it doing its job," says Raymond. "Now we eat for our bodies to be fueled, not to be stuffed. It's weird to think we were once so into fast food. It was our thing."

Throughout this book, I've told you the stories of a lot of different people with the goal of helping to inspire you. They're not offered, though, for you to compare yourself to them. Comparing yourself to someone else can sometimes motivate you, but it can also help you spiral downward, negating all the gains you make. Your journey is *your* journey. We have to drive home this point on our shows since people are losing weight in a group. Mostly, being in a group is great—that's why I've been encouraging you to reach out. A group gives you a platform for sharing ideas, and there is built-in support. But if group members compare themselves to one another, it can get ugly.

You don't even have to be in a group to get depressed because someone lost more weight than you, or that you lost weight but didn't end up looking like a movie star. Compare yourself to only one person: you. Have you done amazing things? (Yes.) Are you staying on target? (Hopefully.) Life is unfair. People are going to do things better than you, get more breaks than you—you can make yourself crazy looking at the inequities in life. I'm not saying a little competition isn't good. We created a whole show—*The Biggest Loser*—based on that premise. But mostly in life, if you want to keep the weight off, be competitive with yourself. Each week, do better than the next. Set new goals. Try new things. Don't stand still.

Here is something else that can help. Don't be alarmed if you don't feel comfortable in your new body right away. "It was a hard adjustment," admits Jen, the woman whose 7,000-calorie burn I told you about earlier. "I felt comfortable being heavy, hiding behind my weight." After she lost 66 pounds, people began to look at her, something she found hard to get used to. Many people feel this way; the trick is to not let it send you back to the refrigerator. Talk to someone about your feelings and give it time. You will get used to the new you soon enough—and so will everyone else.

CHAPTER 20

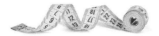

Pass It On

Embarking on a journey to change your life requires that you be self-centered, at least for a while. But, when you've achieved your goal, the beauty is that you get to help other people follow suit. You get to pay it forward.

When we created shows like *The Biggest Loser, The Revolution,* and *Extreme Weight Loss,* our ambition was to not only get a cast full of people to whittle down their bodies but to show the world that anyone who sets his or her mind to it (and gets some help) can achieve remarkable things. Sure, lots of people watch transformative weight-loss shows because they're rubberneckers; they want to see some disasters. But most people want to be inspired—and they are. We don't know how many viewers have been motivated to begin their own weight-loss journey after viewing an episode of one our shows worldwide, but we know that there is a big ripple effect. Many viewers embark upon weight-loss journeys of their own after watching one of these shows. That's one of the greatest rewards of producing them. And to think that when we first started *The Biggest Loser,* I was just hoping to get viewers to order the side salad instead of the french fries and to actually go to the gym instead of hitting their snooze buttons. Who knew we were about to start such a movement?

|||||||||||||||||||||||||||||||||||||||||||||||||||||||||||||||||||||||||||||

It Goes Beyond You: Your Weight Loss Will Inspire Others

JD,

It has been an incredible year for both me and my family. *Extreme Weight Loss* has forever changed my life, and I thank you for choosing me! I have been given the most incredible gift a person can receive—my life! This past year has changed my focus, my purpose, and most important, my life. *Extreme Weight Loss* has also changed my family. My wife has lost 50 pounds, my mother lost 72 pounds (at age 70), and my son lost 35 pounds!

—Bob, *Extreme Weight Loss* cast member, via email

And we know that the audience ripple effect is only part of what gets sent out into the world post-airing. Most of the cast members leave the show determined to help others do what they have just done. They not only want to give back but they know that they have a wealth of knowledge to share. They know, too, that helping someone else helps them stay accountable. I eat better when I'm helping someone change their diet because I know they're watching me (and I want to practice what I preach).

There are so many different ways to help someone else. Pick a person at the gym to help. Offer assistance if you see someone struggling (obviously you have to gauge someone's openness to help, or else you'll just seem annoying). Maybe you'll find a way to help through your work; a lot of former cast members have become trainers or motivational speakers. After Amber lost weight, she was eager to get back to her job at a health-care organization that focuses on preventive health. While she was still heavy, whenever she gave talks about health to groups, she'd always sit behind a table to hide that she wasn't necessarily taking her own advice. Now, thinner and confident that she was on the right track, she returned to work happy that she could speak without hypocrisy and share what she had learned. Some of the people on our shows, including Bruce, have had offers for speaking engagements left and right. Their stories are so inspiring. Your story can be equally inspiring. Remember what Bruce said: "The only thing in life that is not hereditary is your attitude." So change it today and start living the life you know you are capable of living.

I really believe that the goal of the whole weight-loss process is to become a better human being. None of us lives in a vacuum. It's so much easier to live a healthy life when those around you are in step. Many people who've come on our shows lose the weight because they want to be there for their families, and set an example for their kids. One of the most heartbreaking things about finding out that Jeff and Juliana, the father-daughter team we spied on, were lying to us was that the father was essentially giving his daughter permission to be dishonest to herself and everyone else. Luckily, he was able to right that wrong. And look at the role model Jen became for her son when she did the 7,000-calorie challenge. Her son will never forget that night or the lesson that you can do anything you set your mind to. Like I always say, **kids won't listen to a word you say, but they watch everything you do.**

One of the many people I know of who has paid it forward is Josh, a guy that, as you might remember, wasn't even on the show. When Josh was trying to lose weight on his own, a trainer of a gym he belonged to took him on for free. Now Josh is a personal trainer himself, and he takes on some clients for no charge, too. Probably what's even more important, though, is that he counsels them to believe in themselves because that was the magic ticket that lead to his own success. And he doesn't let people get away with anything. He posts things on his Facebook page like, "Feel like giving up? Don't! You are so much stronger than you ever imagined." and "If it is important to you, you will find a way. If not, you'll find an excuse."

A former cast member named Melissa is someone else who paid it forward in a big way. One of the things she remembers most about her stint on *Extreme Weight Loss* was the totally unexpected help she received from people in her town. Melissa came on the show as a widow and single mother. Her husband, a recent army veteran with post-traumatic stress syndrome, took his own life, leaving her with two broken-up kids and in-laws who blamed her for not preventing her husband's death. "Crying into her Nutella," as Melissa put it, she ended up at 301 pounds.

At one point during the show, we asked Melissa to run ten miles. At the time, it seemed like an impossible task. How was she going to do it? She asked people in her Ohio town for help, and a woman named Deanna came out of the woodwork and said, "I'll help you." Deanna became Melissa's running coach and, later, the two of them formed a workout group called Twisted Sisters.

"I wanted to form a workout group but Deanna said, 'I'm a runner; I don't work out.' I'll teach you, I told her," says Melissa. "I had had five stomach surgeries, so when I first started trying to lose weight, I couldn't do a single sit-up, but by then I could bust out 50 of them." The two of them invited five other women to join them. Melissa knew that feeling of walking into a gym, seeing bouncy 20-year-olds working out on the exercise machines at level seven while she was at level two, crying, and then walking out. She wanted to pass on an important lesson she'd learned: The only person you need to keep up with is yourself.

Once the word was out about Twisted Sisters, it grew to 60 people in one month. And women continued to come in droves. Did I mention that Melissa and Deanna conduct the workouts daily—for free? The group participates in 5Ks and is known for doing Indian runs, borrowed from Navy Seal training. About 20 of them run in a line holding a rope above their heads as, in rotation, the person at the end of the line sprints to the front. They've caused such a sensation (and raised a lot of money for different 5K causes) that organizers are lining up to get them to participate in their races. Knowing that all these women are counting on her, Melissa *has to* keep working out. No wonder she's kept off most of the 142 pounds she lost on *Extreme Weight Loss*. She's given back, while continuing to get something, too.

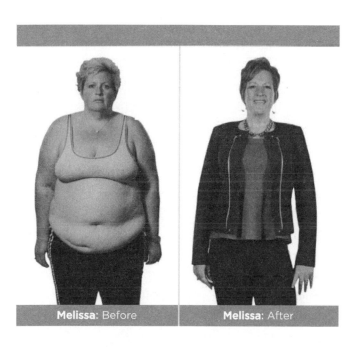

Melissa: Before   **Melissa**: After

What is life really about, if not service? Giving back warms the heart and keeps the fire in our bellies. We are not selfish creatures put on this Earth to be alone. We need to share experiences and feelings, including our pain, with others. As we inspire each other, we create bonds that no one can break. Don't strive to be perfect. Strive to be connected. Connected to other people, your own family, and to yourself. If you can't love—truly love—yourself, you will never be able to love others. You are special; we all are. Remember what I said earlier: Ordinary people do extraordinary things every day.

‖‖

Helping Others Is the Icing on the Cake

Hi,

I remember being in every interview leading up to the interview with ABC execs, thinking, "How am I still here? I have no crazy tragic story to tell or skeletons in my closet to release." I was the way I was solely because of myself and my poor decision-making skills when it comes to good judgment.

With that being said, I have spent my entire adult life in this body. I've been wallowing in my own self-pity, because I was stuck in this rut, and I didn't know how or where to begin just to get out of it. I fought for years to figure out who I am and what my purpose on this Earth was supposed to be, since I'm the one who has to live this life.

Now I know exactly who I am and what my worth is. I am here not for myself, but for the people around me. I'm here for the girls who write me constantly to tell me that they admire what I'm doing and look up to me. I love inspiring other people, because that's what gave me the lift and confidence to get to the point I'm at today. I love the fact that I get to inspire so many known and unknown people. It's extremely scary and humbling at the same time.

—Brandi, *Extreme Weight Loss* cast member,
via email

Scientists have done a lot of research on the people who live the longest. One of the longest-living cultures resides on a small island near Greece. It has more people living over 100 years old then anywhere in the world. When asked what are the top reasons they live so long, the three answers that come back are: 1) Sharing their harvest with the rest of the community; 2) walking each night to meet in a center square for discussions with neighbors; and 3) being connected to other people in the village for survival.

Do you see a common thread in all three? Emotionally connect to your community and the people in it. If one person suffers, we all suffer. People looking out for each other, helping each other, and supporting each other. I want to live to over 100, so I am trying all of these things. And even if I only live until 99, it feels good to help others and see the smiles on people's faces when you do something for them that they didn't expect—and without wanting anything in return.

As you help others, I also want you to spend more time on yourself, even if it means working harder so you can leave work 30 minutes early three days a week to do something for your health (I know, it sounds like a lot to fit in, but you can do it). Be bold. Make decisions that inspire you. Challenge yourself. Turn the TV off for a solid week and see how much extra time you have to improve your life. If you are on medication, realize that within 30 days of eating right and exercising, many medications are not needed. Don't assume once your doctor gives you a pill, that you are now a patient for life. (But remember to check with your doctor before stopping or changing any medications!) Grab control of your life. After all, you only get one, so live it without regrets.

Let me leave you with these parting thoughts. Losing weight is all about changing your mind-set and searching your soul. Determine what you want out of life, then go get it! Don't let a defeatist attitude or buried secrets stop you. Don't be a victim. Deal with the emotional aspects of your life that need attention and fight each day for what you want. Because you are worth it. Say it out loud!

"I'm going to fight each day because I am worth it!"

Say it a thousand times a day until you believe it. Because I already do. I believe in you. I know the power of your mind, and I know you are capable of anything.

APPENDIX

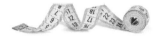

Thirty Days to the Life You're Dreaming Of

What's easier, taking multiple pills each day or working your butt off exercising and eating right? A pill, of course—the pharmaceutical industry is counting on you to say that! Their quarterly earnings depend on it. But if everyone chose exercise and a nutritionally rich diet instead, many people could live a life free of pills. The most underused antidepressant on the planet is a pair of running shoes!

I've seen people go off medication after a mere 30 days of exercise and eating healthfully. No more insulin, no more blood pressure medication, no more Prozac and Xanax, no more Lipitor . . . the list goes on. Even if you're not on medication, isn't your quality of life worth 30 days of hard work? Thirty days is the perfect amount of time to get control and launch you into a totally new lifestyle. Thirty days to help you feel alive again. Thirty days to teach all those naysayers to be proud of you.

Don't get me wrong. You can't just go back to your old ways after 30 days. But 30 days will give you a jump-start, a path into a whole new way of living. What follows are a month's worth of ideas to help you put all that I've talked about into practice. There's a sort of order to them, but you can really do them in any order. Just do them! That's all I care about.

As you go through the next month, there are a few things I think will increase your chances of success. The first is, start your day by doing something good for yourself. Exercise is my number-one choice for starting the day, because if you don't get it out of the way early, you have a greater likelihood of just saying "forget it" later in the day. But if you're not a morning exerciser, then start the day with a healthy breakfast. None of the bear claw pastries, fast-food breakfast sandwiches, or triple-mocha-latte crap. Start out eating something good for you at the beginning of the day, and chances are that you'll make smart food decisions the rest of the day, too.

The second thing I would advise you to do is surround yourself with people who will cheer you on, help you, inspire you, hold you accountable—and just hold you if you need a hug. Everything I've set out for you in this 30-day plan will work so much better if you have like-minded, compassionate people by your side.

Remember, this is just 30 days to get you going and help you try out some new ways of living. Don't take your foot off the gas after 30 days—or anytime in the future. You're in this for a lifetime!

DAY 1

Just Take a Walk

That's it. Take a walk. Don't run before you can walk. Literally. Start with something you know you can accomplish: Go for a 30-minute walk after dinner. Don't worry about speed; don't worry about distance. No data other than time. Just walk. Go out 15 minutes, come back 15 minutes. Now from this day forward, do this every night. If it's not safe for you to walk at night where you live, do it on your lunch hour or some other time of day. What you want to do is create a habit. Maybe you did something similar with your kids or your parents did it with you: Every night, there's bath, books, then bed. It's a habit, routine. Walking is going to be the same thing for you. Don't deviate, just like you don't deviate from brushing your teeth each night. This is a very simple way to start training yourself to live differently.

Ultimately, you should use these walks to segue into a more vigorous cardiovascular workout routine. This could be anything from more walking to running or working out on an elliptical trainer. Get that heart rate up! Check back into Chapter 16 to help you think about the options open to you.

DAY 2

Wake Up to Your Body

Just how hungry are you? Probably not as hungry as you think. I'm going to take a wild guess and say that you like to pile up your plate high. And maybe once you've stuffed all of that food down, you even feel pretty uncomfortable. "Oh, I ate too much!" Still, you do it again at the next meal, and the one after that. You have to wake up to your body. There's a reason your eyes are bigger than your stomach. It takes time for your brain to get the signal that your stomach has had enough. If you keep eating without pause, you're never going to get the message, and you're never going to retrain yourself to eat moderate amounts of food.

Today, you're going to prove that you don't need the piles of wings and mountain of pasta you think you do. Make up your dinner plate as you normally would. Dish up the vegetables, put some chicken beside it, spoon on some rice—whatever you usually eat when you're trying to eat healthfully, and however much of it you usually eat. Eat half of it. Take your plate into the kitchen, and go for the 30-minute walk that's now part of your regular routine. If you're still hungry after the 30 minutes are up, eat the rest of the food. Most people never do.

DAY 3

Upset Your Grocery Cart

Not literally, of course. You don't need to do anything that radical. Nor do you need to go home and start throwing out everything in your refrigerator, freezer, and cupboards. Again, let's take it a step at a time.

We are all creatures of habit. We go to the same seven places; we eat the same seven foods. Our grocery store rituals are embedded in our psyches. We're all always grabbing the same stuff—it's one of the hardest habits to break. If the same stuff were always, say, broccoli, carrots, strawberries, fish, whole-grain bread, a bag of beans, and almonds, that habit wouldn't be a problem. But, of course, you know and I know it's not.

Now you're going to do things a little differently. The ultimate goal is to greatly reduce how many highly processed, packaged foods you eat. And by that I mean things like crackers, cookies, soups (other than low-sodium broths for cooking with), salad dressings, ketchup, frozen pizzas and taquitos, sugary cereals, sweetened yogurts, pasta mixes that come in a box . . . you get the idea. Reducing your intake of these types of foods alone will cut your calorie intake, not to mention the amount of sodium, chemicals, unhealthy fats, and sugar you eat.

Start by doing your regular shopping and choosing the things you usually do (buy small amounts so you can use them up quickly and move on to healthier eating). Count how many packages are in your cart versus the number of produce or meat/poultry/seafood bags (frozen food bags only count if you have healthy frozen fruits and vegetables or lean sources of protein like fish in them). Write it down. Twenty-five packaged goods, three bags of fruits and vegetables, one bag from the poultry department, whatever. Give yourself a pass for things that come in a package but aren't highly processed such as whole wheat bread, corn tortillas, low-sodium beans and low-fat and low-sugar condiments like salsa and mustard. Then, the next time you go to the market, try to shift the balance. (Better yet, now that you have your package count, put all that stuff back and start over.) If you have 25 packaged goods, try to get it to less than 20 items, replacing them with foods like tomatoes and peaches or other in-season fruits and vegetables from the produce section. The next time you go, get it to less than 15 packaged items. Keep going every week and, before you know it, you will have totally transformed your kitchen without even trying. You'll also have transformed your mind-set. "I don't eat (many) packaged foods!"

DAY 4

Turn "I Can't" Into "I Can"

It bears repeating: There are two types of people. Those who say they can and those that say they can't, and both are right. You're about to gradually become an "I can" person. Use today to start counting how many times a day you say "I can't." It doesn't have to relate to eating or exercise. Maybe you say things like, "I can't finish all these dishes tonight, I have to go to bed" or "I can't face looking at the want-ads even though I know I need a new job." It could be anything, big or small. And it's not just the things you say out loud. The voice in your head can be very negative, too—sometimes even more so. More often than not, that voice in our heads has power over us we are not even aware of! Just count how many times you stop yourself from doing something because you don't think you're capable of it. I bet it will be more times than you think.

Tomorrow, start replacing one of those "I can'ts" with "I can." If you counted seven "I can'ts," knock it down to six. Reduce the number the following day, then again the day after that. See how far you can go with it. Train your brain. You think you can never avoid the cupcakes they bring in for birthday parties at work? Try it. Tell yourself, "I can avoid them," then watch yourself succeed.

Better yet, put that cupcake on your desk, right in front of you. When your co-workers come by and ask why you haven't eaten it yet, say, "Because I own that cupcake's ass!" Eventually, smash it with your fist and toss it. (Do not lick that fist!) Make it an event! Tell the whole office at the exact strike of 5:00 p.m. I will smash this cupcake with my fist! See! You can do it. If you say "I can" to yourself multiple times a day, seven days a week, pretty soon that is going to be your go-to place. Any time a challenge comes up, your response is going to be, "Yeah, I can do that."

DAY 5

Partner Up

Over the last few years, something has come to light about people who live well into their 90s and even to 100. Yes, most of them are physically active; yes, most eat a primarily plant-based diet and consume neither too much food nor too little; and yes, most get enough sleep. But what really stands out in my mind is that all of them have a sense of community. They reach out to other people.

All throughout this book, I've been urging you to find like-minded comrades. Today I want you to identify someone—or several people—that you can exercise with. It can be a spouse, your child, a neighbor, a friend, a relative, even just an acquaintance that you think would be willing. This is going to allow you to kill two birds with one stone. On the one hand, you'll get out and move because there is someone there to hold you accountable (just as you are there to hold the other person accountable). On the other hand, this is going to give you the opportunity to add that all-important social factor to your day.

And, believe me, it can end up being a very deep connection. There is something about the mix of endorphins and conversation that leads people to confide in one another. I have had exercise partners tell me things so private, they haven't even told their wives. Think of today's strategy as fostering the sociability factor you need to live longer *and* potentially giving you the emotional release you need. As I've been drilling into your head all along, the emotional component of weight loss is so important—more important than what type of diet or exercise you choose. If you can find someone to talk to during this time when feelings seem to naturally bubble to the surface, it's going to help you in your quest for a healthier body.

DAY 6

Record Your Victories

I'm as big a fan of the grand gesture as the next person (the proof is in the 7,000-calorie burn), but I'm an even bigger fan of dreaming big and racking up small victories. Little acts of courage are performed every day, yet often go unnoticed. I think they mean something, and there's no doubt that they add up and can even inspire you to do bigger things (like a 7,000-calorie-burn challenge). Here's what I want you to do. Keep a log of your little victories. Write down three things each day that you accomplish. Nothing is too inconsequential. "I went to the gym even though I didn't want to." "I paid all my bills." "I took care of that huge pile of laundry that was covering the floor of my bedroom." "I turned down a slice of my mother's famous chocolate cake." Go back and read your log periodically. How are you doing? How far have you come? Don't underestimate the importance of writing your victories down. It only has to be a few sentences a day, but putting a date stamp on it will serve its purpose six months from now when you look back and see how many successes you've racked up.

DAY 7

Take a Lunch "Break"

Like most people, you're probably used to gobbling up your lunch in ten minutes, then lounging around for the remainder of the hour. Here's a way to use your lunch more constructively. When I say take a lunch break, what I really mean is break up your lunch. One season, we made our cast members walk three miles to Subway, the sandwich shop. They were probably happy to have arrived, but before they could get too complacent, we told them they were only getting *part* of their lunch—to get the rest, they'd have to walk to the next Subway, another three miles away.

You may not have the luxury of getting six miles in during lunch, but on days when you're going out for lunch, you can still break it up. Buy an apple at one place, then walk to another place (no, not the place next door—make it as far away as you can reasonably fit into your lunch schedule) for your sandwich, then another place for your drink. If you don't work in a place where you can walk restaurant to restaurant, or if you're brown-bagging it (always a good way to control your calorie intake), break your lunch break in half: Spend half the time—or less—eating, then spend the remaining minutes going for a walk.

DAY 8

Get into the Compliment Business

We spend so much of the day beating ourselves up for what we haven't done or couldn't achieve that we never stop to show ourselves some love. You are a good person, and it's necessary to stop and remind yourself of that. Today, stop yourself five times and give yourself a compliment, a pat on the back for something you did that was worthy. "Nice job on not eating that cupcake." "You were awesome at work today." "You were easygoing when that guy took your parking space." "You took a walk during lunch." It could be anything; just take the time to acknowledge it.

Today, when negative thoughts come, and they will, replace those with love. So today it's not, "I can't believe I'm so fat" or "I hate myself because I have no willpower"; instead, it's "I am a strong person who can overcome adversity" and "I am a good person who has done good for others." Give yourself the love, forgiveness, and encouragement that you give other people, and amazing things will start to happen.

Most of the overweight people I've met over the years have a very difficult time giving themselves compliments. They find it easy to pat someone else on the back but get queasy when it comes to praising themselves. It's not vain to do so! Don't spend your time being hard on yourself; that's just going to lead to a pity ice-cream party. Spend some time loving yourself, and you'll want to treat yourself well, not spite yourself by eating junk food and sitting immobile on the couch.

DAY 9

Everybody Needs a Mantra

Working out is hard; making the right decisions about food is hard. But what if you had a thought in your head that got you past the difficulties? It would almost be like having someone looking over your shoulder, urging you on, and making sure you're going in the right direction. That's what a mantra is. It's a reminder, a go-to line that swims around your head providing encouragement and reinforcement.

Today, you're going to start putting your mantra into play. When you think you can't do that last rep or push-up, when you hear that bag of salt-and-vinegar potato chips calling your name, pull out that mantra. What should your mantra be? If there's some quote you've heard that speaks to you, make it your mantra. Or create your own. There are no rules. Here are a few that might work for you, too:

- Whatever you put into it, you're going to get out of it.
- Today's going to be the hardest day ever, but it's going to be a great day.
- The only thing in life that isn't hereditary is your attitude.
- I made a promise to myself, and I'm keeping it.
- Fall down five times, get up six.

One of my favorite mantras was one used by a cast member named Rod. Whenever he was wavering on working out or about to cheat on his diet, he'd say to himself "Can't go back. . . . Won't go back. . . . Not this time." He even got it tattooed on the inside of his forearms.

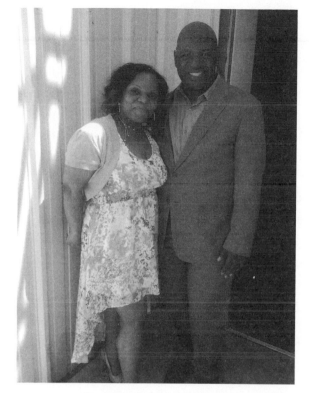

Rod with his cousin Anika

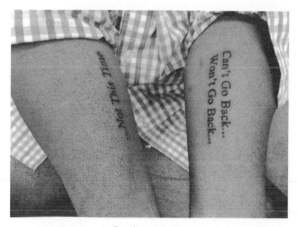

Rod's mantra

DAY 10

See It, Believe It

When everyone around you is enjoying pizza and beer, ordering the salad and sparkling water feels like punishment. When you just got off work and would like nothing better than to go home and get in that recliner with your laptop and a glass of wine, going to the gym can seem like too big a pain in the butt. But your butt is exactly what's at stake. So remember why you're doing this. Go into your closet and pull out that pair of jeans that hasn't fit you in years, and bring them out. Now hang them somewhere in your bedroom so that every time you walk in, you can see them. Leave the jeans there as a constant reminder of your goal. We once had someone on the show that hung the dress she wanted to wear on her refrigerator. Every time she went to get something to eat, she *had* to make the right choice. Maybe a little over the top, but a good idea.

DAY 11

Move More During the Day

By now, you probably have noticed people wearing bands around their wrists that don't quite look like watches, but don't quite look like bracelets either. These fitness trackers are great for letting you keep track of how much you move per day (obviously with the goal being to burn more calories), but you don't need a fancy fitness tracker to get an idea of whether you're getting up and around enough.

Today, using a stopwatch or the stopwatch function on your watch or a step counter app on your phone, track how much time during your day you spend walking around, climbing stairs, just getting from place to place. I'm not talking about working out; just your regular daily movement.

What I like about logging your progress is that it turns into a little competition with yourself. Can you do more than the day before? Can your weekly tally beat the previous week? Trust me, charting your movements is going to make you want to move more. It also gives you clues for how to improve on what works for you. Add it to your daily routine.

You can also make it into a little competition with your mate, friends, or co-workers. Bet them that your weekly combined movement will be more than theirs, and report your totals to them every day.

DAY 12

Show Your Co-Workers You Mean Business

The workplace is the worst place for people who want to lose weight. There's always some guy who thinks he's being generous by bringing in doughnuts every Monday morning. Then there are the group lunches ordered from fast-food places; meetings with frothy, fattening drinks; and the big bowl of candy sitting on a well-meaning (but clueless) co-worker's desk. Today, you're going to fight back by arming yourself with the right stuff. Bring an apple or other healthy snack to a meeting. Everyone else will be envious of your willpower and forethought, and the snap of the apple as you bite into it will get everyone's mouth watering. (Bring an extra one and give it to the person who comments first.) Brown bag it even if you know the boss is springing for pizza in the conference room. Stock your desk drawer or locker with nutritious foods you can turn to when the office vending machine beckons. The message here: Be prepared!

There's also a kind of built-in bonus to showing such discipline at work. It will show your boss that you are in control of your life, which can be a good career move. Being in control is powerful, and powerful people usually get paid more!

DAY 13

Take the Candy Bar Challenge

Say you unwrap a candy bar, break it in half and set it out where you can see it oozing caramel and peanuts (or whatever your candy bar of your choice features). If you had cameras on you, it would keep you honest. Nobody wants his or her weakness to be public knowledge. But if you're in a one-bedroom apartment and that candy bar is sitting on the coffee table where you typically put all of your take-out food, the voice in your head telling you to grab and eat it is going to get very loud. (By the way, even skinny people hear that voice; they just don't put themselves in a position to have to fight it.)

Now take a photograph of that oozing candy bar and post it on Facebook with a sentence about how, in a test of willpower, you're not going to eat it for 24 hours. Then report in. "Four hours down." "Fifteen more hours to go." You'll get comments like, "Oh my god, I could never do it!" and "You go, girl."

This small exercise is going to make you feel empowered. And how great will it be when, at the 24-hour mark, you post a picture of yourself tossing that candy bar in the garbage? (Let me just add that, as a precaution, pour soap over that candy bar. I've had people tell me that they've dug food out of the garbage.) You might even take a video of yourself running over the candy bar with your car. Post the video; people will love it! I would definitely give it a "like" if I saw it.

DAY 14

Talk, Talk, Talk

When you feel yourself wavering in the face of temptation today—or maybe you already made a mistake—call someone, preferably someone who's been through it themselves, and talk about it. What do alcoholics do when they are on the verge of screwing up? They call their sponsors. That's because a sponsor is not going to judge you; a sponsor has been there. Their job is to help you and make you feel good, not shame you so that you spiral into a binge. This is the same thing.

Talking about it will keep shame from creeping in. Shame is worse than the cupcake. Giving your feelings a voice by sharing them with others turns the volume of shame down. This is an effective tool to keep yourself on task. When your shame volume starts to creep up, stop eating and start talking!

Even if you don't have a friend or family member who has struggled with weight to call, choose someone who can be honest with you. You don't want your go-to to be someone who's going to pat you on the back and say you did a great job when you didn't. It has to be someone who will say something like, "Okay, you made that mistake, now move on," or, "Okay, you're feeling temptation, everyone does, but you made a promise to yourself." A big part of your assignment in this weight-loss journey was to enlist support—now use it!

DAY 15

Play with Perception

In my household, we eat our dinner on salad plates. I'm no saint: If I had a regular-size dinner plate, I'd fill it up just like everyone else. Nobody wants to see a little circle of rice surrounded by blank space; it makes you feel like you're being punished! It's human nature to want to fill up the plate. I used to do it all the time, and the upshot was that I'd end up eating a giant bowl of pasta and other outsized meals. But then we decided to change our serving routine. We started using the salad plates. And guess what happened? Our portions came down to a healthier size. But, and this is a big "but," we didn't feel deprived. We felt satisfied even though we were eating less, because our plates were empty when we were finished. Just another mind trick!

Maybe you've heard this change-your-plates tip before, but believe me, it really works. That's because we're not really hungry for everything on our plate, but we eat it anyway because it's there. It's Mount Everest. It's there, we climb (eat) it. If you're using smaller plates and bowls, you'll still eat what's there, but it will be less—though your brain won't register that. It's all about perception. We think we're so smart, but we're easily fooled! Today, give it a try. Even if you do go back for seconds, you're going to end up eating fewer calories.

DAY 16

Keep Promises to Yourself

Today we're going to work on keeping the vows you make to yourself. How many things have you been promising yourself that you're going to do, only to back out again and again? Today (and the day after that and the day after that) is going to be different. And just to be clear, when I talk about keeping your promises to yourself, I don't mean *kind of* keeping them. Go the whole way. If you say you're going to eat a healthy lunch, don't order a turkey sandwich with mustard, then grab a bag of potato chips at the register. Get in the habit of keeping your promises to the letter.

As with everything, go for reasonable, not radical. Don't promise to do an hour of cardio if you haven't exercised in a year; unless you're walking, that's overreaching. So to begin, make a list of your promises for the day. Things like, "I promise to do 30 minutes on the treadmill." Again, that does not mean you get off at 25 minutes or even 29 minutes, no matter how much you want to. If you write down 30 minutes, do 30 minutes! Believe me, your body will send powerful signals telling you to get off early, but if you stay with it, eventually your body will get accustomed to the challenge and reward you for finishing.

Also, don't underestimate what you are capable of. If you start with 30 minutes of walking, add 5 minutes a day after that. Remind yourself it is only a number. That number cannot beat you, only *you* can beat you. Plenty of people I work with on my shows say "I could never run at a 5.5 pace on the treadmill." To prove them wrong, I put a towel over the readout, slowly move the pace up to a 7, and they don't even notice! So don't let a number put a glass ceiling on your progress.

DAY 17

Skip the Package Deal

On Day 3, I had you revise your shopping list, reducing the number of highly processed packaged goods you throw into your grocery cart. Let's build on that. A lot of the packaged foods people eat don't come from their kitchens; they come from vending machines, the well (but toxically) stocked break room kitchen at their work, a quick duck into the mini-mart when they stop for gas, and so on. This goes for restaurant meals, too, since who knows what's really in them? It's not in your control.

The easiest way to gain control of what you put in your mouth is to decrease those packaged/restaurant meals. I'm not suggesting you never eat out. But I am suggesting that you reduce eating out as much as you can. If you always buy lunch at the corner deli, try brown-bagging it, and I bet you'll lose five pounds—if not more. It can make a real difference—you'll see.

How many packages do you open in a day? Just like you did on Day 2, do a count, then incrementally reduce the number. You eat ten a day, next week eat eight. Keep going from there.

DAY 18

The Top-of-the-Hour Workout

Today is all about getting active, really active. At the top of every hour, 9:00 a.m. to 5:00 p.m., I want you to do either five push-ups or run up one flight of stairs. Think about it. Five push-ups might take you 15 seconds, but if you do it at the top of every hour, you will have done 40 push-ups for the day! And running up a flight of stairs takes less than 10 seconds, but at day's end, you will have done about 8 flights. That's pretty amazing.

Do this every day for 7 days, then add a push-up or flight of stairs for the next 7 days. Keep adding until you're ultimately doing 8 push-ups or 4 flights eight times a day (a total of 64 push-ups or 32 flights daily). I guarantee you will feel the benefits big time. Chances are, you'll draw others in as well. I did the push-ups challenge at my office and by the week's end, there were nine of us doing it. At the top of every hour, we'd all run out of our offices, meet in the hallway and get our push-ups on. It was incredibly fun and gave us all a much-needed energy boost. The shared camaraderie of a stunt like this can really bring people together, too.

DAY 19

Get the White Out

Nutrition rules keep changing all the time. First fat's bad for you, then it's good for you. Don't eat eggs. No, eggs are okay. Carbs are the way to go. Oops, we mean protein. It gets confusing. Still, I think if you just use common sense, you'll know that no good is going to come of living on bacon and pork ribs. I think it's pretty clear now, too, that a diet made up almost wholly of foods collectively know as "white foods"—pasta, white bread, white rice, crackers, and most cereals—will make you fat and damage your health. For instance, it's known that refined foods are stripped of fiber, one of the elements of food that helps you feel full. Refined foods also raise blood sugar, triggering the release of insulin. Both things can make you feel hungry and crave more calories Plus, white foods are mostly empty calories—you get very few nutrients from these foods—and many of them contain high fructose corn syrup, which has been linked to obesity and diabetes.

Today, take all of the white foods I named out of your diet. Nothing white except cauliflower. I think you're going to actually find that you feel good. Try it again for another day, and another. See where you can go with it, how long you can last. You'll be on a streak! "I haven't eaten white foods for two weeks." Not wanting to break the streak may actually lead you to a healthier diet.

DAY 20

Do What You Have to Do (First)

Do what you *have to* do, before you do what you *want to* do. I say this to my kids every day. "Dad, let's play basketball!"

"Did you do your homework?"

"Not yet."

"Okay, do your homework, then we'll play ball."

Doing what you have to do before you do what you want to do is a philosophy of life that can help you head in the right direction. Working out, eating right, getting your life in order are the priorities to put at the top of your list. Then do things that you want to do like watching TV, going online, sleeping in. It may seem unrelated to weight loss, but it's all a part of reorganizing your life for the better. Today, as you go about your day, keep that adage in mind, and catch yourself when you fall off the path. Ask yourself: *Did I do what I had to do before I started to do what I want to do?* Then make sure the answer is yes.

DAY 21

Go Commercial-Free

How much TV do you watch? Don't even answer that because whatever it is, it's too much! Odd words coming from a television producer, I know, but even I know that TV can be a time suck that prevents you from doing healthier things. And, most likely, consciously or unconsciously, you associate watching TV with eating. Super Bowl Sunday and cheesy nachos, binge-watching *The Walking Dead* and binge-eating mint chip ice cream—they go together like salt and pepper. And what else is the Food Network for if not to inspire you to eat? Likewise, commercials can propel you right into the kitchen either out of avoidance or because the bacon cheeseburger being advertised has you salivating.

So let's begin there. Today, when you watch TV, do not watch a *single* commercial. Instead, get up and move. Every one-hour show has 18 minutes of commercials; if you watch two hours of TV without moving, that's 36 minutes of exercise that you're losing out on! Make it heart-pumping and nonstop for the whole break—jumping jacks and squats are always good. The next time there's a commercial break, change it up, maybe do some push-ups and sit-ups. The time after that, do burpees (the exercise where you squat down, place your palms flat on the floor, kick you legs back, then pull them back to the squatting position; repeat) or run up the stairs. The choices are endless. Keep it interesting!

And what if you've DVR'd your show or are watching premium channels without commercial interruption? Create a rule for yourself and set the timer on your phone: every half hour of binge watching you'll stop and take an exercise break.

DAY 22

Break the Fast-Food Habit

There is a reason so many people turn to fast food for the majority of their meals, or even just some of their meals. Actually two reasons: It's cheap, and it's convenient. This is something you already know. You also know that fast food—and let's be honest, you probably don't order the salad or any of the other healthier options some places now offer—is the worst thing for your health and your waistline. You have to cut it out of your life.

You don't even need to know much about cooking in order to break the fast-food habit. And the thing is, it's actually not that much more work—and it's even cheaper—to just buy a rotisserie chicken at the market, a bag of corn tortillas, a can of beans, some lettuce and tomatoes, some broccoli, some olive oil and vinegar. Right there, you have two nights' meals: chicken, salad, and broccoli one night; chicken tacos and beans the next.

If you're industrious, you can even use the leftover chicken carcass to make chicken soup. (All you do is add water and some chopped celery and carrots and boil for a few hours.) Cut up some extra carrots and celery instead of steaming broccoli, and you won't even need to use your stove on night one. Just be a good shopper, and you'll never use the excuse "I can only afford fast food" again!

DAY 23

Put a Positive Spin on Things

One of my sons is really into golf, and he watches this great motivational video that I think also has a good lesson for anyone who wants to accomplish anything. When most golfers take a bad shot, they typically curse at themselves and, say, "That was the worst shot," or, "I suck at golf," then they move on to the next shot. That just reinforces negativity. What you want to do instead is reinforce positivity. Here's how the video advises that golfers do it: Every time you take a shot you say, in your head, "great shot," "good shot," or "needs work." Just a simple (but not downbeat) assessment of how you did. Then, before you move to the next hole, you take a practice swing and say to yourself, "great shot."

Sounds stupid, right? Who's going to pat themselves on the back like that? But then I thought about it. What you're doing by rating your shot, then taking another stroke and saying "great shot" to yourself is training the pathways in your brain. You're erasing the bad shot from your consciousness. When the last thing you hear is "great shot," it seeps into your brain, setting the stage for actually making a great shot the next time around.

One day, it occurred to me that this technique could help with weight loss. So, today, try this. Step on the scale and look at the number. Then say to yourself, "great week," "good week," or "needs work." Then step off the scale, look at it, and say, "great week." The last thing your brain hears is going to be overwhelmingly positive. Now see if you can capture that feeling again—this time for real—next week.

I know this exercise (and some of the others in this plan) may seem silly, but they have been tested over and over again, and they work. So don't just read them, think "that's cute," and go on to the next page. Really try them, stick with it, and enjoy the results!

DAY 24

Find the Hidden Sugar

I want to prove to you that life can be sweet without sugar. I'm not saying that you should never eat foods that contain sugar, but I think you'll find that once you reduce the amount you eat, you'll crave it less and end up eating fewer "empty" calories overall. Today, grab a notebook and go on a sugar scavenger hunt through your refrigerator and pantry to see how much sweetness is lurking. There may be the obvious things, i.e., cookies, ice cream, certain cereals, and so on (though I hope you've got all those obvious sweets out of the house by now). But I also want you to look for less obvious sugary foods, things like ketchup, BBQ sauce, salad dressings, Chinese sauces, pasta sauces, fruit yogurt, energy drinks, and even seemingly healthy things like dried fruit (when the fruit dries up, the sugar concentrates). Check labels for dead-giveaway ingredients: honey, brown sugar, turbinado, molasses, high-fructose corn syrup, other syrups, raw sugar, agave and glucose (including other sweeteners ending in "ose"). Now that you know where the sugar is, work on working it *out* of your life.

It may take a little sleuthing, but grocery stores do stock versions of these items without the added sugar. Another way to avoid these sugar traps is to make these foods from scratch. You will be surprised how easy it is to make salsa, salad dressing, and many sauces with no sugar—and by how much better they taste, too!

DAY 25

Take Your Intensity Up This Week by Doing Cardio Intervals

By now, I assume (hope!) that you're well into a cardio workout routine. Now it's time to start bumping it up. Intervals—pushing your pace up, then slowing down to recover so you can speed up again—help you burn more fat in less time.

In 2008, researchers at the University of New South Wales, Sydney, Australia, had a group of women ride stationary bikes at intervals of 8 seconds sprinting and 12 seconds slow riding for 20 minutes (60 repeats in all). The researchers then compared them to a second group of women who rode for 40 minutes straight at the same speed only to find that, at the end of 15 weeks, the interval trainers lost more weight and more body fat than the steady riders. The only question is, Why would you *not* do intervals?!

Target certain days of the week for interval training—maybe do it Monday, Wednesday, and Friday. Then experiment with different equipment to see where you are really enjoying the workout. I personally enjoy doing intervals on a treadmill way more than on a stationary bike. Try everything until you find your sweet spot!

DAY 26

Be a Stand-Up Guy (or Gal)

Sitting, it seems, is the new smoking. Even if you exercise for an hour or more a day, according to new research, it doesn't cancel out the bad effects of sitting the rest of the day. That was a rude awakening! I was working out hard in the morning, then sitting at my desk all day. Had to change that. Standing more won't necessarily help you lose weight, but it will, by all accounts, help extend your life. That may be why you hear a lot now about people buying stand-up desks to help solve the sitting problem. You don't, though, need a sophisticated system. That all goes back to excuses. If you want to stand more while you're working, put a large, weighted box on your desk and place your computer on top.

That's not going to work for everybody, but there are lots of other ways to make sure you stand more and sit less. On Day 11, I gave you a strategy for moving more. Starting today, work standing into it. Now, as soon as I get an email, I delete it, get up, walk to the person's office, then stand while talking to them. I stand when I talk on the phone. When there's a crowded room, I let others take the chairs and stand up instead. At my kids' school, they now break every 15 minutes to stand up and shake out their bodies. Set your watch or phone to remind you to do the same. And next time someone offers you a seat, say "no, thanks."

DAY 27

Take a Time Out

One of the reasons it's so easy to get off-track is busyness. Running here and there, constantly consuming information—our lives are chaos. It's exhausting just to keep up, and so much easier to let your guard down and go back to your old bad habits if you feel overwhelmed. Today, I want you to begin doing something that I have started to do recently, which is meditate. But let's not even call it meditation, which might be too out there for some people, and let's just call it a daily time out. It's a chance to go inward for a time and re-center yourself so that it's easier to stay on track. And it's therapeutic. Letting one thought roll into another thought; you don't know where it's going to take you. Ultimately, I've found that if you can work up to even just 15 to 20 minutes, it can have a similar effect to exercise, where endorphins kick in and you feel almost as though you're floating.

Here's an easy way to try it out: Put the distractions away and just sit on the floor comfortably. Pick a spot to look at, and don't look away for five minutes. Let your thoughts come, one thought rolling into another thought. The meditation expert I've worked with gives these guidelines: If a thought about the past comes up, let the "movie" play with no questions; anything about what's happening around you currently—for instance, thoughts about sounds you hear in the distance or how your body feels—go with it; but any thoughts about the future, shut them down. Those are the kinds of thoughts that bring on anxiety and worries. Instead, bring your mind back to your breathing, to the spot your looking at, or to any thoughts that don't concern the future.

Negative thoughts are going to come in. Let those thoughts wash over you, and realize that no one is perfect. We are all a work in progress—which means you will get there, a little at a time, not all at once. Try to love yourself more, and when negativity creeps in, try to match it with love for yourself. Stay positive. You are a good person, who does good things. Visualize something you did that mattered and felt good. In most cases while meditating, I try to keep my mind open to whatever pops in and learn from the way meditation floats you in and out of certain moments. Good thoughts or bad, you will learn from both.

This is just one type of meditating. There are many types, and you can find many good guided meditations on YouTube. I urge you to explore until you find something that resonates with you, and to make a concerted effort to have a point in the day when you go inward, even just for a few minutes. You'll see what a calming effect it can have. Keep in mind, too, that you may have to work up to sitting for an extended length of time. It's like exercise—you don't go out and run six miles right off the bat. You start with a block or two and increase your mileage over time. Same with meditation; you work up to it. But even if the very idea of meditation is daunting don't give up on it: Even sitting in a room in complete silence for 2 to 3 minutes can have a calming effect.

DAY 28

Get Your Game On

Not long ago, I got an email from a former cast member of *Extreme Weight Loss* named Patrick. "Hey, JD!" he wrote, "I came out of Thanksgiving day great! I took a food scale with me to measure my protein. Did not have mashed potatoes, stuffing, or rolls. (Did have just a smidgen of pecan pie.)"

That was all great—I was proud of him. But what really piqued my interest was what came next: "I also took a deck of cards and every 20 minutes [had] someone draw a card that corresponded to an exercise I had to do. For example, the 5 of hearts was 5 burpees; 8 of diamonds, 8 push-ups . . . and, yes, I did do them! Even got the kids involved. They were doing the exercises with me. Most successful Thanksgiving I've ever had and never one moment felt so stuffed that I was miserable."

Is that a great idea or what? Today, or, if need be, next time you are in a social situation or having a family dinner, I want you to try this. Don't wait for Thanksgiving. This is a fun game that can help you get a little exercise in while also helping to take the focus off food. When you have a healthy and amusing diversion like Patrick's game, who needs something sedentary like Scrabble?

DAY 29

Find a Challenge

Having a goal in front of you can help you stay focused and motivated. It's true of any endeavor, but especially true of exercise. Make your workouts count for something. Today, start looking online or checking local sports stores for upcoming events you can train for. It doesn't have to be a marathon; it can be a 5K walk.

And don't freak out if it's billed as a race. I have a slogan I use with cast members on our shows: Don't compete, just complete. When we'd sign them up for events, they'd say things like, "I can't compete with all those athletes." That's not the point. The point is to just cross the finish line. Your only competition is you. When you show up at the event, keep that line in your head: "I'm here to complete, not compete." That's going to prevent negative, shameful thoughts from popping into your mind and prevent you from quitting. All you need to do is finish—no matter how long it takes. And when you do, congratulate yourself on keeping your promise!

DAY 30

Be Honest and Relax

Going forward in the weeks and months to come, there are two things that I believe will help everything fall into place: One is being honest with yourself and others; the other is relaxing. It sounds kind of corny, but those two things provide a foundation for healthful living—for everything, really. If you're honest with yourself—Did I do my best today? Did I keep my promises?—and honest with others—I'm having a hard time today; I could use some help—then you can just relax. And by relaxing you are taking away all of the stress that can send you straight into self-destructive mode. Constantly freaking out over whether you're following every dietary rule perfectly doesn't help you. Knowing that you did your best on a given day—or admitting to yourself that you didn't—will free you to move forward. That's why honesty is so important. If you don't beat yourself up about asking for help or having a cookie, you can chill. Slow life down a little bit. Get off the hamster wheel. When you do, it's easier to get things done in a positive way.

These are two simple concepts, but they're not always easy. I'm great with the honesty part; I have to work on the relaxing part every day. Whichever way it plays out for you, don't give up. Lying and stressing out make people fat. Honesty and relaxation make them thin, healthy, and, most importantly, happy. I know you'll prove me right!

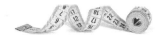

Resources

You know how I feel about excuses: they're inexcusable! Maybe the worst excuse of all, though, is that you don't have the knowledge you need to lose weight. Well if you don't have it now, it's easy enough to get. Good health information is out there all around you so don't try playing the "I don't know how" card as a justification for staying fat.

The list that follows includes documentaries, books and websites that can all help you understand where you're going and how to get there. These are things that have swayed my own thinking on nutrition, fitness, and overall health. I hope they influence you as well.

Documentaries

All of these movies really changed how I look at food. They all basically arrive at the same conclusion—that the American diet needs to change—though they each come at it from a different angle. They are all also straightforward, research-based, eye-opening, and even life-changing.

Cowspiracy: The Sustainability Secret —Looks at the devastating environmental impact of factory farming.

Fat, Sick & Nearly Dead—Australian Joe Cross crisscrosses America with a juicer in an attempt to lose weight and regain his health (spoiler alert: he succeeds).

Food, Inc.—Journalist Eric Schlosser, who wrote *Fast Food Nation,* (see below) made this film about the corporate-controlled food industry.

Food Matters—A documentary about the reluctance of the medical community to acknowledge the benefits of food as medicine.

Forks Over Knives—Explores the premise that many chronic diseases can be controlled and even reversed by eliminating animal and processed foods.

Hungry for Change—An indictment of the diet industry's deceptive tactics.

PlantPure Nation—Nelson Campbell, son of the nutrition research pioneer T. Colin Campbell, puts a plant-based diet to the test by trying it out on a North Carolina rural community raised on comfort foods. Good health ensues.

Super Size Me—See what happens when director Morgan Spurlock lives on a diet of food from McDonald's for a month (it isn't pretty).

Books

This lineup of books provides everything from information on the science of nutritious eating to inspiration for living a healthier, happier life.

Born to Run: A Hidden Tribe, Superathletes, and the Greatest Race the World Has Never Seen by Chris McDougall—Even if you never plan to run a day in your life (and could care less about athletics), this book will inspire you to take on challenges. It tells an amazing true story and offers a great lesson to anyone needing a kick in the butt.

Fast Food Nation by Eric Schlosser—This expose of the fast-food industry will make you think twice before breezing through the drive-thru. Schlosser was one of the first people to give us a behind-the-scenes look at the companies contributing to obesity in America.

Plant-Based Diet for Dummies by Marni Wasserman—Educates on the "whys" and the "hows" of adopting a plant-based way of eating. A great way to get started.

The China Study: The Most Comprehensive Study of Nutrition Ever Conducted and the Startling Implications by Thomas Campbell and T. Colin Campbell, M.D.—Chock full of science, this is not an easy read, but it's worth the effort. Dr. Campbell is my idol; he is the Michael Jordan of nutrition.

The Prophet by Kahlil Gibran—I read this when I was in my 20s and try to pick it up every few years as a spiritual refresher.

The Road Less Traveled: A New Psychology of Love, Traditional Values and Spiritual Growth by M. Scott Peck, M.D.—An oldie but a goodie, this is one of the first self help books to ever hook me in. Life is difficult, and this author doesn't try to play that down. Instead, he writes about the process of searching for and confronting what causes your unhappiness.

How Not to Die: Discover the Foods Scientifically Proven to Reverse Disease by Michael Greger, M.D., and Gene Stone—A doctor explains how nutrition and lifestyle choices can literally save your life.

Cookbooks

Don't think that because you start eating well, you'll never get pleasure from food again. These cookbooks prove that the right kind of cooking can keep you both healthy and happy.

Deliciously Ella by Ella Woodward—The author of this book was sick and her doctors were having trouble finding a cure. Taking matters into her own hands, Ella adopted a plant-based, gluten-free diet and immediately became better. She shares her simple but delicious recipes here.

Forks Over Knives The Cookbook: Over 300 Recipes for Plant-Based Eating All Through the Year by Del Sroufe—Filled with recipes that are easy to make, practical, and have no added oils. Most fats from these recipes are derived through nuts, seeds, or avocado. Don't knock it 'til you try it!! They are delish!

Plenty More: Vibrant Vegetable Cooking by Yotam Ottolenghi—So many brilliant primarily plant-based recipes (with gorgeous pictures). Most of the recipes are a little more involved, but worth it.

River Cottage Veg by Hugh Fearnley-Whittingstall—A chef famous for meat in England takes a turn for the healthier. These creative recipes feature all different types of grains and vegetables. We've made many things out of this cookbook for dinner parties to rave reviews.

The China Study Cookbook(s) by Leanne Campbell—These are a series of books that take up where the film *Forks Over Knives* left off. The recipes are oil free, very practical, and very tasty.

The Plantpower Way: Whole Food Plant-Based Recipes and Guidance for the Whole Family by Rich Roll and Julie Piatt—Rich Roll has a great story. He was a middle-aged guy sitting in an office chair all day practicing law. He realized he was feeling terrible and decided to get himself in shape. He's not a guy who does things halfway, so he started with long-distance running and very shortly made his way into doing grueling ultramarathons. He discovered plant-based eating fueled him the best. He shares his recipes, created with his wife, a chef, in this book. His memoir *Finding Ultra* is one of my favorites as well.

The Plant-Based Journey: A Step-By-Step Guide to Transitioning to a Healthy Lifestyle and Achieving Your Ideal Weight by Lani Muelrath—If you could use a very specific plan for changing your diet, this is it. The author includes meal plans and easy recipes.

Thug Kitchen: The Official Cookbook: Eat Like You Give a F*ck by Matt Holloway and Michelle Davis—These guys are hilarious. The recipes in here are as creative as they are delicious and the delivery is, shall we say . . . unique.

Websites

You really don't have to go further than your computer to get good nutrition information and lots of delicious recipes. Here are the websites my family frequents (and one my wife, Chrissy, produces—the first one is her blog).

plantbasedluv.com

nutritionfacts.org

forksoverknives.com

engine2diet.com

ornishspectrum.com
(Dr. Dean Ornish's program to reverse heart disease)

pcrm.org/health
(The Physicians Committee for Responsible Medicine)

thugkitchen.com

Acknowledgments

If the root of transformation is desire, where does that desire come from? I would have to first give the credit to my parents, who always taught me that if you want something, you should stop talking about it and go do it. Take action. To my dad who puts loyalty and hard work above all other virtues. A man who tried to keep me humble by reminding me, "I don't care how famous you are, there are like a billion people in China who never heard of you. . . . Now go take out the garbage." To my mom, whose support for anything I wanted to achieve in life was limitless. She protected me from all things evil. To my twin sister, Heidi, whose ability to nurture has made her a superb pediatrician and a great friend, and my "little sis," Alison, who put up with me using her head as a kick ball when I was 12. To all of you, I say, love you guys, and thank you for being my family.

For the last 23 years I have had a best friend who knows no limitations and whose ability to love me unconditionally has taught me more then anyone I have ever met. Chrissy, I owe you everything. From the moment I laid eyes on you, I knew I would look into those eyes for the rest of my life. If something special happens, it doesn't *really* happen until I tell it to you. You make everything real. Chrissy, you constantly inspire me to be a better person, husband, father, friend. I still can't believe you agreed to marry me, and I wonder every day when you will finally turn to me and tell me it was all a big mistake. I am more in love with you now than when we first met, especially after you read this book and told me you loved it. Being a physical therapist has lead to your (our) passion for eating healthy, and living a fit life, and I am so glad it is a priority for our family. Your tireless work of keeping all your boys happy does not go unnoticed. You're our queen, and all three of us look at you like you're the most beautiful woman on the planet inside and out. And you are.

My boys! Cooper and Duncan. The two best kids a dad could ever ask for. Watching you live a passionate life is a gift that never gets old. As I have told you a million times, the only thing that is measured in life is the size of your heart, and you both have immeasurable hearts. Being proud of you everyday is a feeling that will never get old. Keep living a life full of giving to others and helping to make this place we live in better. And thank goodness you both look like your mom.

My business partner of 25 years and counting, Todd Nelson. Without you, buddy, the hits don't happen and the creativity disappears. You have been by my side since the early days, in the foxhole together, and have never wavered once. The unspoken commitment we have towards each other will never be professionally equaled. Personally, you are the brother I never had, and I will always remember ever, battle we won, everyone who tried to take us down, and most of all, in those moments where our company, or a show, or both were in peril, I knew I could always turn my head, look at you, and together we would figure it out and come out on top!

To my running group of nearly a decade, I owe you all a debt of gratitude for not only showing up in the dark most mornings, but for sharing your innermost thoughts, feelings, and personal life stories. You all keep me fired up about running, life, and always trying to be the best athlete I can be. I feel lucky for knowing all of you, and don't take lightly the bond we have all created over the years. And out of 12 people in the group we are still ALL married and believe in the work it takes to stay that way!

To Bob Harper and Jillian Michaels. If we never found each other, I truly believe *The Biggest Loser* would not still be on television today. You both taught me so much over the years, and your commitment to excellence is unmatched. You two are the reason that show worked, and I will forever be grateful that you came into my life. Some things are just meant to be.

To the Season 1 contestants of *The Biggest Loser*, we all went on a journey that included bumps, bruises, tears, and more than a little yelling, but it ended in creating a movement for change. You were pioneers along with me in the journey to demand a better life. No short cuts. No cutting, stapling, or sucking, just good old-fashioned hard work. It started a revolution and changed the way America looked at what was possible. We learned as we went, and inspired each other to keep going. It wasn't easy, but we used every obstacle as an inspiration and along the way helped reshape what America thinks about change. You were first. You had to blaze the trail for what would become one of the most successful television franchises in history. I thank you for everything and wish you and your families only the best.

For the past half decade, Chris and Heidi Powell, you have traveled the globe preaching the gospel of healthy living for *Extreme Weight Loss*. You both work yourself into exhaustion, giving until it literally hurts, with no boundaries other than helping anyone who wants help. You are both 360 degrees of love and passion for always doing what's right, and never leaving anyone behind. First class in every category, I have so much respect for your commitment to do the job right. You practice what you preach, and it is refreshing, even after half a decade, how you will both go the extra mile for a contestant, even at the personal sacrifice of your own health. May there be many more successes in your future, because they are well deserved.

To my place of worship . . . the Steve Mareska gym, my place of spiritual guidance. I look to you as my guru on all things in life not just how to stay fit, but how to live a full life. You are a leader, a good human being, and the spirit lift I need every time I am lucky enough to be around you. You are also very bald, but I won't hold that against you.

There was one guy when I was thinking of writing a book who said the simplest two words I ever heard. They were also the words that got me to sit down at the scary blank page and begin to write. Those words were. . . . "Why not?" Idan Ravin, whose own book, *The Hoops Whisperer*, is inspiring all by itself, made me want to put my passion of transformation on paper. Thank you for staring at me with those piercing, intense blue eyes and saying, "Why not?" That long pause after you asked me that question was fear. How could I write a book? Talk, yes. I can talk all day to anyone who would listen. But write? Then, like I tell everyone I work with on the weight-loss shows, I remembered my own mantra. Fear is good. Lean into it. Embrace that feeling and turn it into action. So, the next day, I sat down and started to write. . . . *Todah,* my friend!

Daryn Eller, you are a fantastic collaborator. You always made me feel like my voice mattered, helped give me a POV, and beyond being a terrific listener, you are a good soul. As you know that means more to me then any resume or college attended. I felt that the minute I met you. Thank you for helping me make this dream a reality, and helping me to find a voice to convey such an important message in this book. I hope this experience was as rewarding for you as it was for me.

Hanzy baby, my oldest friend, college roommate, agent, confidant, and lover of all things that drive, your support to help make my dreams come true since I met you in 1986, as a teenager at USC, on my first day of college has been one of the luckiest things that has ever happened to me. We had no cell phones, computers, or apps for finding the perfect college roommate, we just got lucky. You were with me, before I was me. You were there when I got my big break as host of Fox's *Fun House,* and when it hit as the #1 kids' show in America. My life changed forever. From a college campus sophomore, to the cover of *Teen Beat*, through it, our friendship only grew closer. You were right there at the start of my company, which went from Todd and me on my front porch to one of the largest independent production companies in the world, and even helped me set meetings for this silly idea I had to write a book. At every major point in my life, you have been there to support me, make me laugh, and break bread. I hope I have been able to reciprocate in some way for how you have made me feel over the years. In life, they say we are lucky to maybe have one lifelong friend. Between you and Todd, I am blessed to have at least two.

Kurty B, my other brother I never had, I learned more from you about how to conduct myself in the television business then anyone else I have ever known. Your brilliance is obvious even though you are the only man I know who can turn 5 hours of work into a 12-hour day. To your defense, it is the greatest entertainment a day could be filled with, ever. And to your best friend growing up, Scott Edel, who has been my lawyer and integrity compass for the past 25 years, I thank you for always being there to support and guide me, and to remind me that good guys can finish first. Mark White, or Whitey, as I have been calling you for the last 25 years as my loyal friend and advisor. You have always been genuinely happy when something good happens to me, and I will always consider your family my family. Mama D, my #1 fan, I will never stop appreciating the love you always show me for everything I try to accomplish.

My editor, Andrea Au Levitt, I can still hear the excitement in your voice the first time we spoke on the phone, which fed my enthusiasm to try to deliver the best book I had in me. Thank you for always being open to listen, decisive in your opinion, and willing to try all. It's rare for someone in your position to give a first-time writer so much room to either fail or succeed and continue to lead them toward success.

To all the people that agreed to bare their souls on one of our transformative TV shows, and in this book. You are brave men and women, who looked fear in the face and ran toward action to change! You were willing to expose your lives, warts and all, share your innermost personal stories with courage and compassion, which is rare to find these days. Those stories continue to inspire me, and millions of viewers all over the world, as an example of someone who demands more out of their lives. To live longer, with more quality, and to love yourself unconditionally. We are all human, so there will be mistakes made, cookies eaten, and weight gained and lost, but ultimately it is not the falling down that now defines you. . . . It's getting back up time and time again, to take back control, and kick shame's ass! I have hugged all of you at one point when I could not get my arms around you, and then again at the end when my arms wrapped all the way around until they were touching on the other side. You have loved me, hated me (sometimes both in the same day), but ultimately we have respect for each other. I thank you for helping people overcome issues in their lives, because they saw that you did it in yours.

Index